The
BEAUTY
DIET

The
BEAUTY
DIET

UNLOCK THE FIVE SECRETS OF
AGELESS BEAUTY
FROM THE INSIDE OUT

DAVID WOLFE

With R. A. GAUTHIER

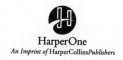

HarperOne
An Imprint of HarperCollins*Publishers*

HarperOne

HarperCollins books may be purchased for educational, business, or sales promotional use. For information, please email the Special Markets Department at SPsales@harpercollins.com.

FIRST HARPERCOLLINS PAPERBACK EDITION PUBLISHED IN 2020

Designed by Ad Librum

Library of Congress Cataloging-in-Publication Data is available upon request.

ISBN 978-0-06-230981-5

20 21 22 23 24 LSC 10 9 8 7 6 5 4 3 2 1

This book is dedicated to
the Immortal Spirit of Beauty.

Contents

The Five Beauty Factors

I believe the pursuit of beauty is a noble one—our appearance is a mirror that reflects who we are, revealing our lifestyle choices, our state of mind, and our potential.

Everyone wants to feel beautiful. You've picked up this book because you too seek lasting, sustainable beauty. Unfortunately, it is the desire to *be* beautiful, instead of to create, feel, and nourish beauty, that has fueled the 160-billion-dollars-a-year beauty and cosmetics industry and created a culture of comparing, criticizing, correcting, concealing, and camouflaging.

We cover our bodies with products labeled "natural" that actually contain dangerous ingredients. Of the 82,000 chemicals used in beauty and cosmetic products, most of these include carcinogens, reproductive toxins, hormone disruptors, and pesticides. On average, women in the United States use 12 personal care or cosmetic products a day, which can contain 168 different chemicals. Teens are exposed to even more chemicals; they use on average 17 products per day. And although men use fewer products, they still are exposed to 85 different chemicals. Every. Single. Day.

The way we go about being beautiful is woefully misguided. This onslaught of toxic chemicals, preservatives, pesticides, heavy metals, and harmful electromagnetic frequencies pollutes our bodies, accelerates our aging, ravages our complexion, and destroys our energy and vitality, effectively un-beautifying us. Then we are forced to seek solutions for our early aging symptoms in the bottles of more cosmetic and beauty products, creating a vicious cycle of toxicity that not only empties our wallets but also keeps us from attaining the beauty we so desire.

I have spoken to tens of thousands of women from all around the world at my events, book signings, retreats, and lectures, and what has shocked me most about the pursuit of beauty is how dissatisfied nearly all women are with how they look and feel. *Did you know that only 2 percent of women consider themselves to be beautiful?* I've learned firsthand through these conversations the immediate and long-term consequences of the fear-driven cosmetics and beauty business that preys upon women's insecurities and feelings of inadequacy. The women I've talked to share feelings of disempowerment and are victims of a collective brainwashing. They are forced to believe that beauty is determined by a number on a scale, the size of their waist, the shape of their butt, and the voluptuousness of their lips.

As a result, women are willing to submit to increasingly riskier cosmetic procedures, from tummy tucks to face-lifts, Botox® injections, butt implants, and breast augmentations, all in an effort to attain the "ideal" beauty, which is an airbrushed illusion in the first place. In fact, many women who attend my lectures seek my advice on how to *reverse* the damage the surgeries, procedures, and chemical peels have done to their faces and bodies.

Essentially, we have, as a society, removed Mother Earth from the beauty equation. We have become mistrustful of and embarrassed about our bodies, feeling disappointed and betrayed by them, when, in fact, nature has created perfection in each and every one of us. All we have to do is let that shine through. We have sought solutions from a synthetic, human-made, chemically driven cosmetics culture that destroys our health and our environment when the solutions to our problems are right in front of us.

The ancient civilizations of Greece, Rome, Egypt, China, and India relied upon the natural resources offered by Mother Earth to beautify themselves. We can learn a lot from ancient wisdom and experience. The time-tested beauty secrets I will be sharing in these pages are, in fact, nothing new; they are quite old—centuries old. After returning our faith and confidence to the miracles of nature and ourselves, we can make more informed decisions regarding what to put on and in our bodies.

The path to beauty is simple. When we take cues from our ancestors and tap into nature's abundant resources, we can experience optimal health on every level, which in turn allows us to exude both inner and outer beauty. Now is the best time ever to take advantage of what Mother Earth provides. We have unprecedented access to the purest and most potent superfoods, superherbs, medicinal mushrooms, and unique plant oils from around the world. Due to extraordinary advances in technology, there are alternatives that, when used in combination with nature's offerings, enable us to bring our bodies back into balance and experience superior health and vitality.

Over the past several decades I have engaged in rigorous study, research, and self-experimentation by incorporating the wisdom of the ancients with the bounty of the earth. In this book, I will share everything I have learned with you so you can look and feel the *best* ever. This information isn't complicated, and my suggestions aren't costly or invasive. You don't need face-lifts or fillers to turn back time; you can experience youth, radiance, and vitality by eating life-enhancing foods that create the inner glow that is your birthright.

MY PHILOSOPHY

There are five beauty factors that will lead you to a state of "beyond beautiful"—that is, a state of superior health and vitality from the inside out. These five factors are the foundations upon which radiant health is built. Put simply, if you optimize these factors to suit your individual lifestyle and follow them consistently in your day-to-day life, you will undergo a beauty transformation.

The Five Beauty Factors

1. **Eat for Beauty:** Nutrition is the foundation of beauty. The only true way to maintain supple skin, shiny hair, a joyful outlook, and energy all day long is by keeping a close eye on what you do—and don't!—put into your body. In the "Eat for Beauty" chapter, you will learn how to identify and access the best foods ever and avoid harmful ones from the moment you wake up, from the top ten superfoods and superherbs to the other extreme—the most contaminated food substances passed off as "safe" food. Through powerful nutrition, you can restore, rejuvenate, and activate the natural elasticity in your skin in a way no invasive cosmetic procedure or synthetic beauty product ever could. You will read about cutting-edge research on the benefits of healthy fats and oils, superfood nutrients, mineralization, good carbohydrates, plant proteins, and more.

2. **Remove Toxins:** Toxins are lurking everywhere—in the air we breathe, the homes we inhabit, the food we eat, the water we drink, the clothes we wear, and the many products we put on

our bodies every single day. Over time, all the chemicals we are bombarded with block the body's natural ability to detoxify itself, and we enter into a state of toxic overload. As we become more deficient in essential nutrients and vitamins, we start to experience constipation, poor skin tone, thinning hair, and stubborn fat. In the "Remove Toxins" chapter, you will find easy ways to avoid harmful chemicals and remove toxic buildup. You will discover how every internal organ, from your liver to your kidneys to your lungs, affects your appearance and how to nourish these organs by removing the toxins that harm them. In addition, you will detox your body, your home, and your life. You will read about the foods, herbs, and daily practices that aid and facilitate detoxification, and the new and exciting research on clay, charcoal, infrared heat, and more.

3. **Nourish Cells:** Beauty is truly built at a cellular level, and your ability to replace and repair cells is the defining characteristic of how strongly you are able to maintain your youth. Furthermore, beauty is not predetermined by genetics. Just because your mother or father has varicose veins, wrinkles, belly fat, or cellulite doesn't mean you will too. Instead, genes are largely influenced by lifestyle—the foundation of a revolutionary new science called epigenetics. You will learn in the "Nourish Cells" chapter about using the science of epigenetics to activate the genes that manifest beauty, keep your youth and energy, stop the aging clock, and flip the switch on your appearance. You will become keenly aware of which vitamins and minerals hydrate and support cells, and which foods and lifestyles cause chronic inflammation.

4. **Balance Hormones:** Everything we do influences our hormones. Many of the chemicals found in the world today disrupt and sab-

otage our hormone health, including pesticides and bisphenol A (BPA), and most, if not all, commercial beauty products contain classic hormone disruptors, such as parabens and phthalates, that wreak havoc on the human endocrine system, causing weight gain (especially visceral—and unfortunately visible!—belly fat), estrogen dominance, cancer, and many side effects that destroy our beauty and sap our energy. In the "Balance Hormones" chapter, you will learn all about your hormones and what foods and products disrupt them. You will discover how to avoid common pitfalls and master hormone-regulating concepts that will help instead of hinder you on your path to beauty. You will also discover how critical sleep is to hormone health and beauty.

5. **Overcome Stress:** Daily stress has a powerful effect on our appearance. But it also deeply affects how we *feel*. The chapter "Overcome Stress" uncovers the toll stress takes on your body and mind. You will find out why stress might be the cause of your rapid weight gain, early aging, sleeplessness, mood swings, and more. You will read about stress-busting strategies that will rejuvenate you, including profound silence, breathing meditation, inversions, forest bathing, and more.

By applying these time-proven principles, which incorporate the beauty secrets of Ayurveda and Traditional Chinese Medicine, you will be empowered to make simple food and lifestyle changes that will help you experience the best health ever and feel young and beautiful at any age!

The truth is, you are *already* beautiful—your body has an innate ability to shine. If you give it what it needs, it will take care of the rest. We can regain our confidence both in ourselves and in our bodies as we move toward beauty as a holistic lifestyle choice. By following the formula prescribed in these pages, you will move toward reenlivening all that makes up the experience of you!

The beauty industry depends upon our lacking this confidence. And because we lack assurance in our own bodies, we take refuge in a superficial system that might be good at masking flaws, such as wrinkles, abdomen fat, and puffy eyes, but these flaws are the body's way of signaling to us that we are on a wrong path.

The information in this book is simple and is the *right* path forward. I promise you, by making a few small changes to your lifestyle, you will experience a huge difference in how you look and feel. Here are the amazing benefits you will gain:

- Radiant, glowing, elastic skin, free of acne, rashes, and/or wrinkles

- Healthy weight loss that is supportive of your lifestyle

- Freedom from digestive troubles, such as constipation, bloating, and gas

- Reduced stress levels, managed with tactics like meditation, exercise, and breathing

- Stronger hair follicles and nails

- A healthy diet, rich in superfoods and superherbs, along with access to recipes that increase your energy and vitality

- Restful, restorative sleep that comes easily

- A healthy sex drive at any age

- Regulated hormones that serve you and end insulin resistance, estrogen dominance, and imbalanced cortisol

- Clean organs capable of filtering contaminants from your body in an efficient way

- And so much more!

MY STORY

I am the son of two medical doctors and was literally conceived in a medical library. I, like my mother and father, once believed in the power of modern medicine. I would go to my dad's practice and watch the steady flow of sick people seeking help. Over time, I realized that the medical and pharmaceutical industries rob Peter to pay Paul. Just like the beauty industry today, they mask the symptoms of disease without addressing the underlying causes.

This left a deep impression on my mind, and I began to investigate where to find true health. *What I discovered was the inherent power and abundant healing ability of Mother Nature.*

My close relationship with nature began at a very early age and followed me through my teenage years and into adulthood. I bought some land and became a farmer. At my agricultural research center in Hawaii known as NoniLand, I now grow cacao (chocolate), vanilla, avocado (they don't call me David "Avocado" Wolfe for nothing!), coconut, mango, noni, coffee, passion fruit, macadamia nuts, baobab, star fruit, lychee, longan, the panama berry tree, citrus fruit of all types, tulsi, ashwagandha, jackfruit, durian, breadfruit, black sapote, eggplant, the pau d'arco tree, akee, and more—I often hand-pollinate each vanilla and durian flower. One thing I have concluded from this personal interaction with plants is that they are intelligent, and the information they communicate can make us happier, healthier, and more beautiful.

My beauty and health expertise does not end with plants. I am also a beekeeper. I provide my bees with the best superfoods and super-herbs ever, so the honey they produce is medicinal. In addition, one of my greatest passions is spring-fed water hunting: finding and experiencing clean, fresh, pure water. As you'll learn in this book, toxin-free, properly hydrating water is one of the keys to a beautiful life.

All these experiences helped me grow on both personal and professional levels. I have written several books about the power of plant-based foods, superfoods, and superherbs, and I have had the privilege and honor to travel and lecture extensively, sharing the information I have learned on the subjects of longevity, superfood nutrition, optimal health, and wellness in twenty-nine countries around the world. I have spent time studying with shamans in the rain forests and mountains of Peru, North American Native American medicine women, European and British folk herbalists, fit and beautiful permaculture activists living off the land in Australia, Hawaiian farmers reviving traditional Polynesian ways, leading master herbalists of Chinese medicine, Ayurvedic scholars and practitioners, Rudolf Steiner, with his legacy of spiritual literature, and more. These sources have all shared with me their most powerful ancient, timeless beauty secrets. And although each of their philosophies may differ slightly, there is one truth shared by all: *beauty is a reflection of optimal health on physical, mental, and emotional levels.*

No matter who you are—whether you are a single mom or a celebrity, a farmer or a fashion model, an elite athlete, a weekend warrior, a business executive, a stay-at-home dad, or a teenager—living a nature-inspired lifestyle like the one described in this book will reconnect you with the most powerful foods and medicines on earth and will move you toward vibrant health.

The Beauty Diet reflects my passions. It is the culmination of all I have learned in my travels, my decades of study, and my dedicated research into what causes people to experience the best health *ever*—reflected in their radiant skin and abundant vitality. I cannot wait to share this information with you!

HOW TO USE THIS BOOK

My guess is that you already know some of the information I'm going to share with you. You have probably done some research yourself and/or know me and my previous work on natural health, beauty, and nutrition. While I encourage you to read this entire book from front to back, and in that order for optimal beauty results, I understand that you may be looking for something specific or may be coming to this book with a wealth of knowledge already. For that reason, I've supplied many resources throughout the book to keep the reading experience smooth, engaging, and informative.

Superfoods and Superherbs: If you're looking for quick information on the top twelve superfoods and top ten superherbs for beauty, this chapter begins on page 49 and functions like a manual you can refer to again and again.

Three-Day Beauty Cleanse: If you're ready to dive into a powerful beauty detox, a three-day cleanse begins on page 235, with recipes appearing in the back of the book, starting on page 243.

One-Week Beauty Jump Start: Ever wonder what a perfect week of eating for beauty looks like? Ever wonder what I eat every day? Flip to the One-Week Beauty Jump Start on page 241 to learn more.

Recipe List: I couldn't limit myself to just one recipe section; you'll find detoxifying, cell-supporting, and nutritious recipes in every chapter. Therefore I compiled a master list of the recipes on page 244 for easy review.

Beauty Recipes: From Gluten-Free Zucchini Chia Muffins to a Very Veggie Nutriblast, from tonics to snacks to daily meals, this section begins on page 243.

Glossary: If you're ever unsure of a complicated, fancy term I use (and I use many of them throughout the book), check the glossary on page 289 for a definition.

Index: The chapters are inherently interconnected. For example, some superfoods you'll learn about in the "Superfoods and Superherbs" chapter help to regulate the hormone cortisol, which I cover in great detail in the "Balance Hormones" chapter. However, the index on page 327 will allow you to jump between sections easily if you seek more information on a certain topic.

Are you ready to start living a healthier, more beautiful life? Let's get started!

Eat for Beauty

The subtle energy of your food becomes your mind.
—The Upanishads

I have spent most of my career exploring and explaining the extraordinary benefits of a plant-based and superfood-based diet. "We are what we eat" is a time-tested mantra, and it rings true today more than ever before. Our current food industry is based on economics. The quality of our food and how healthy it is have become less important than profit. Degenerative diseases are increasing at unprecedented rates, and as a population, we are suffering from malnutrition and obesity simultaneously.

A crucial first step in correcting these issues is to open our eyes to the ways the food and beauty industries operate and to sidestep their entire perverted paradigm. Walking in the grocery store is like walking in a minefield. Although there are some good choices available, avoiding the pitfalls takes knowledge and keen discernment. Overcoming the craving for fake flavoring–filled food might be hard, but you can learn to recognize clever marketing and the obvious manipulation of food labeling laws.

It astounds me that people still think "natural flavors" has anything to do with actual food. For example, some orange juice brands contain "natural flavors." What is natural flavoring? It is simply chemical compounds developed in a food-flavoring laboratory that taste like something natural—in the case of the juice, oranges. "Natural flavors" can consist of up to a hundred different ingredients. This is the mechanism by which processed food, containing beauty-killing ingredients such as refined and processed oils, can be altered to taste like anything at all.

Although people can debate the dangers or benefits of flavoring agents, one thing is clear: flavorings are developed to hide what is underneath, which in many cases is nutrient-absent or even cancer-causing ingredients! Food companies have spent millions on this one aspect of food production, and the payoff for them has been huge.

There is little difference between the cosmetics industry and the food industry. Both use the current labeling laws—or lack thereof—to essentially deceive consumers and rake in enormous profits. By opening your eyes to this, you can walk through your grocery store aisles and make much better food and personal care product choices.

BEAUTY IS AN INSIDE JOB

For decades my message, drawn from personal experience, meticulous research, and strong anecdotal evidence, has been very straightforward: *Take the ancestral approach to optimal health and radiant beauty by eating organic whole foods, as close to nature as possible.* Consume a plant-based diet if you can. Incorporate superfoods and superherbs. Avoid genetically modified, chemical-laden, processed Frankenfood.

But I did not always eat this way. Like most American kids, I once ate the Standard American Diet (SAD), which consisted of Lucky Charms cereal; Wonder Bread; pasteurized, homogenized, glow-in-the-dark, larvicide-laden, herbicide-laden, fungicide-laden, genetically modified, hormonally altered milk in a plastic-leaching jug cut with tap water! My parents didn't know any better. I didn't know any better.

On my way toward getting my master's degree in nutrition, I began a journey of upgrading my diet by juicing celery as well as eating whole, natural foods, including cucumber, tomato, and what would soon become my favorite, avocado. Sounds super simple, right? That's because it is! As I gradually decreased the amount of junk I ate and increased the amount of nutrient-dense, organic, unprocessed foods, I started to feel better.

Then I discovered superfoods (way before "superfood" became a buzzword), like cacao, goji berries, coconut oil, and maca. In fact, with many of these superfoods, I was the first person to put them up on the internet! When I started eating these superfoods, there was a definitive shift in my consciousness. It was easier to make healthy food choices because I understood and was experiencing their bene-fits directly. My complexion improved, my concentration dramatically increased, my recovery after workouts was faster, my energy levels were through the roof, and my teeth and gums were healthy. These improvements had me convinced that health and beauty were accom-plished from the inside out—after all, you are what you eat, from your head down to your feet.

Next, I was led to the sacred superherbs: pearl, schizandra, tulsi, and he shou wu. I became a student of Chinese tonic herbalism and discovered the principles of jing, chi, and shen. I started to incorpo-rate them not just in what I ate but also in my philosophy of life. I realized my calling in the world was to educate people on the power of Mother Nature and all her abundant offerings, including the hidden gems that had made such a difference in my well-being. I started lec-turing all around the country and eventually the world, impassioned by my desire to help people look and feel their best ever—every day.

Nature is simple in its complexity. Within one food we can find medicinal polysaccharides, essential fatty acids, vitamins, minerals, flavonoids, proteins, and amino acids—the steadfast building blocks for strong, supple, glowing skin, hair, nails, and teeth. My advice is to let nature do the work for you. There is no need for the human-made, synthetic chemical concoctions that are taking a devastating toll on our health and environment and that are the instigators of aging and poor health.

The industries of food and cosmetics would have you believe there are no natural solutions to any of your problems. I find it strange that not one hospital in the United States has even a single natural treatment for *anything*. Think about that. A mere hundred years ago there were only natural treatments for everything from a headache to wrinkly skin. We may think we have become more sophisticated in our approach to health, but in reality, we have completely lost the plot. Obesity, heart disease, cancer, accelerated aging, stress, and inflammation have reached epidemic proportions. We need to go back to the basics. I assure you, by eating the foods I prescribe in this chapter, you will activate your potential to experience health and vitality on every level.

By relying upon the wisdom of the ancients, we take the guesswork out of what to eat to be healthy and beautiful. We don't have to follow the latest celebrity fad diet, take the most recent magic health bullet, or continue to be bewildered about what to put into our bodies. Instead, we need to give our bodies the foods and herbs that contain high concentrations of vitamins, minerals, enzymes, antioxidants, and that are alkaline and anti-inflammatory. These also support as well as enhance the body's natural ability to look and feel the best ever. I believe that when we consistently eat an optimal diet, we aid the body in replacing cells, optimizing digestion, gently removing toxins, and assimilating key nutrients that cause gorgeous skin, shiny hair, strong nails, and a stunning smile.

BASIC BEAUTY NUTRITION

Beauty nutrition begins with a clear understanding of the role fats, carbohydrates, and proteins play in supporting our health and beauty. The best beauty diet is one where these three fundamental components of healthy eating are eaten in proper proportion. Each one of these pieces of the dietary puzzle has been feared, demonized, or championed at one time or another. With a multitude of dietary paradigms and the experts continuously changing their advice as to the "best" way of eating, is it any wonder that 76 percent of Americans feel it's impossible to know which nutritional guidance to follow? In fact, 52 percent state that filling out their income taxes is more straightforward than trying to figure out what they should eat!

We need to sort through all the conflicting information to understand how to approach these three nutritional categories and *how to apply that understanding to our unique body type.*

Fats, carbs, and proteins are all equally important to the body's ability to express beauty. When you eat too many fats and oils, for example, you can prompt weight gain and heart-related issues, but it's critical to eat enough fat to maintain the elasticity and moisture of your skin. Carbohydrates from real food sources like raw fruits and vegetables make us glow, fueling us with energy to get through our day with their rich stores of vitamins and minerals. Conversely, processed carbohydrates spike blood sugar, cause weight gain, and create inflammation. The right amount of protein, meanwhile, allows us to create the basic building blocks to power our cells, creating soft, supple skin. Too much protein can cause body odor and acne breakouts. When we begin to understand how to consume proteins, carbohydrates, and fats in a balanced, healthy way, they can work synergistically within us to create the most radiant health ever.

Debunking the Fat-Free Scam

Don't be fooled! Beware of foods advertised as "low-fat," "light," "reduced fat," "nonfat," or "fat-free." These words are marketing scams aimed at making you think you are selecting a healthier version of a product when, in fact, the opposite is true. Fat adds flavor. Take away fat, flavor is lost. Therefore fat-free foods are loaded with genetically modified and/or artificial ingredients and chemicals to make up for the loss in taste, such as chemical table salt, sugar, high-fructose corn syrup, modified food starch, maltodextrin, monosodium glutamate (MSG), hydrolyzed vegetable protein, guar, and xanthan. Such ingredients can cause low brain function, gut-related health problems, overeating and weight gain, insulin resistance and diabetes, hormone imbalances, inflammation, and heart disease.

FATS

Fats have been thoroughly shamed in the media, but the truth is we need a healthy supply of them every single day to support our beauty processes. When we eat fat, we are encouraging the growth of muscle tissue, regulating our metabolism, supporting our reproductive health, fighting depression to improve our mood, increasing the strength of our bones, and bolstering our immune system. The brain is made up of and fueled by fat—we literally can't think as clearly without enough of it in our diet.

The body requires fat for long-term energy. It supports the function of our thyroid and keeps our hormones in balance by producing cholesterol, which is critical to healthy hormone production. Fat is one of the building blocks in the body that creates healthy skin and collagen. It protects skin cells from sun damage and hydrates the outer lipid layer of our skin to keep it looking plump and youthful.

When we eat good plant fat we take in linoleic and linolenic acid, which are essential fatty acids (EFAs) that the body is unable to produce on its own. We need these EFAs in order for our joints to remain fluid and for all the tissues in the body to function normally, including our heart. Fat allows us to absorb minerals and important nutrients like vitamins A, D, E, and K properly. The composition of our blood and our body temperature depend on fat to stay balanced and lubricated. When we have fat in combination with a meal, it can bolster weight-loss efforts by keeping us feeling full for longer periods of time.

If fat is so important to overall body function, why is it so frowned upon? The reason can be found in the type of fat we eat—saturated or unsaturated—and the answer as to which is best may surprise you.

Saturated Fat

Saturated fats have been the target of a massive smear campaign since the 1950s, denounced for clogging our arteries, negatively impacting our cholesterol, and causing us to develop heart disease. While there is some truth to this crusade because *some* saturated fats contribute to these problematic conditions, *other* saturated fats beautify our skin, lubricate our joints, keep our mood stable, contribute to the health of our bones, and make up 50 percent of our cell membranes.

Scientifically speaking, when a fatty acid has all its available carbon bonds connected to hydrogen atoms, they pack together tightly and become highly stable. Because of this, saturated fats don't go rancid easily and they become solid or semisolid at room temperature. It's important to understand that while good saturated fats like coconut oil raise our LDL (bad cholesterol), they also raise our HDL (good cholesterol), and the ratio of the two to each other is a much stronger predictor of heart disease and cardiovascular problems than anything else. Bad sources of saturated fat, like commercially raised red meat and dairy products and commercially prepared baked goods, that raise only our LDL should be avoided at all costs. The saturated fat in a drive-through cheeseburger is destructive, whereas the saturated fat in coconut oil is critical for bodily functions.

Monounsaturated Fat

These fats lack two hydrogen atoms in comparison to saturated fats. This means they don't pack together as tightly, are not quite as stable, and tend to be liquid at room temperature. Olive oil is a prime (and very delicious) example of a monounsaturated fat. It's best to pour this type of fat on top of your food rather than cooking with it as heat can make it rancid.

The best monounsaturated raw food sources: almonds, avocados, cashews, durian, olives, pecans, and stone-crushed oils.

Polyunsaturated Fat

This type of fat lacks four or more hydrogen atoms, making it highly unstable and prone to high rancidity. If we look to the past, our ancestors ate a high amount of saturated and monounsaturated fat in the forms of lard, tallow, butter, and olive oil. The rate of heart disease was almost nonexistent then. Fast-forward to today and almost 30 percent of calories in the average American diet come from processed polyunsaturated fat like vegetable oil derived from soy or corn, or from safflower and canola oil—and heart disease is running rampant.

These types of polyunsaturated oils oxidize quickly when exposed

---

Durian

I am a huge fan of this "stinky" fruit. It looks like a hedgehog, smells like rotten onions, but tastes like heaven to me! You will either love it or hate it. There is no middle ground with durian. Considered to be "the king of fruits" in Southeast Asia, durian is packed with vitamin C, which fights free radicals, reduces oxidative stress, and slows down aging. Durian also possesses strong beautifying characteristics including a high concentration of raw oleic fats, vitamin E, sulfur compounds, and soft proteins. For a fruit, durian actually contains a high concentration of protein, with 1 to 2 grams per section of the fruit.

---

to heat, oxygen, and moisture, which most often occurs during processing, but can also happen while sitting on the grocery store shelf or when cooked in food. Once they go rancid, polyunsaturated oils contain free radicals. Every time we eat these free radical–filled oils we increase our risk of liver damage, digestive problems, immune system dysfunction, and reproductive damage. We are subjecting ourselves to DNA/RNA strand damage; impairing our brain function; causing wrinkles and premature aging of the skin; damaging our tissues, organs, and blood vessels; and sparking weight gain.

To make matters even worse, most polyunsaturated oils contain a very high level of omega-6 fatty acids and very few omega-3 fatty acids. These omegas are best kept in balance, and when we have an abundance of omega-6s in our food we mess with our prostaglandin production. This disruption can create blood clots, high blood pressure, inflammation, weight gain, and decreased immune system function.

We do have the choice to enjoy quality polyunsaturated fat sources that come from nature, though, and they can be beneficial to our overall health and beauty.

The best polyunsaturated fat raw food sources: borage seed oil, chia seeds, hemp seed oil, hemp seeds, flax, flaxseed oil, primrose oil, and walnuts.

(Note: It is important to keep these oils in dark containers out of direct sunshine and only use oils that have been cold-pressed, not heat extracted.)

Hydrogenation

Hydrogenated oils are free radical–filled, polyunsaturated fats that should be liquid at room temperature but go through a chemical process to alter their form. Tiny metal shards are added to the oil, along with starch and soap-like emulsifiers. The mixture is steam cleaned, and then dye and flavor are added. We end up with compressed blocks of margarines and shortenings.

The way the hydrogen atom moves during the process described above straightens out the molecule, and we call this resulting creation a trans fat. Trans fats are 100 percent toxic to us, but unfortunately the body doesn't recognize them as such. The cells take them in as if they were properly constructed saturated fats and incorporate them into the cell membranes. These Frankenstein fats disturb the chemical processes of the cell going forward, leading to high cholesterol, cardiovascular difficulties, and other long-term illnesses.

Trans fats are even worse for you than regular rancid polyunsaturated oil. Please avoid them at all costs! Seek out extra-virgin olive oil and coconut oil instead.

CARBOHYDRATES

Carbohydrates (sugars) are one of the most misunderstood, yet critically important, parts of a healthy diet. Our cells *need* sugar as fuel. It just has to be the right *type* of sugar—meaning the carbohydrate sugar from an apple is not the same as the carbohydrate sugar from a donut.

The proper carbohydrates not only fuel us with energy, but also keep our weight in check, contribute to a healthy heart, keep our digestive system moving, regulate our insulin and cholesterol, power our muscles, uplift our mood, increase our focus, and enhance our overall beauty and health. The wrong carbohydrates can do the complete opposite by robbing our pancreas, adrenals, and bones of vital minerals; making our skin look puffy and pale; slowing down our brain function; and causing us to gain weight.

So how do we know which carbohydrates we should and should not eat? The answer lies in the type of carb and where we source it from.

Carbohydrates are made up of carbon, hydrogen, and oxygen, and depending on how these elements are arranged, they build single or double sugar units known as "simple carbohydrates" (monosaccharides and disaccharides), longer sugar chains known as "complex carbohydrates" (polysaccharides), and indigestible complex units (fiber).

All carbohydrates get broken down by the body into monosaccharides—single sugar units—because this is the form the body uses for energy. Muscles (including the heart) and the brain require a steady stream of sugar for continuous function. It's not practical to eat constantly, and so the body stores carbohydrates to be used for ongoing muscular activities in the liver. What isn't stored moves into the bloodstream to support the mitochondria in creating nucleotides (ATP and GTP), which fuel cellular activity.

Simple Carbohydrates

Simple carbohydrates like glucose, fructose, sucrose, galactose, mannose, and ribose (note the telltale "ose" at the end) are already monosaccharides and are easiest for the body to absorb and digest. We have the choice to eat natural sources of simple carbs (unrefined) or processed ones (refined). Both types raise our blood sugar swiftly when we need quick energy, as they can enter the bloodstream within minutes. The difference is in their nutritional value.

Unrefined Simple Carbohydrates. Unrefined simple carbohydrates like raw organic fruits, wild fruits with seeds, and honey contain high amounts of vitamins, minerals, and antioxidants. Fruits have the added bonus of being digested more slowly due to all their natural fiber, which helps stabilize blood sugar levels and control appetite.

Refined Simple Carbohydrates. Refined simple carbohydrates are processed foods. Because of the temperatures used during processing, they lose all their naturally occurring healthy elements like fiber, minerals, and vitamins. Oftentimes they end up filled with chemical preservatives and additives as well due to chemical processing methods. Refined carbs can not only damage our internal organs but can contribute to major health concerns like obesity, heart disease, and cardiovascular problems. Eating refined carbs results in higher spikes in blood sugar and, due to the chemicals in them, they are addictive for our body and brain. I'm talking about things like enriched cereals, white bread, white rice, pastries, white flour, pies, cakes, and so on. A good rule of thumb is if it's in a package, avoid it.

Refined sugar is one of the worst possible carbs and I could write an entire book on how destructive this substance is in the body. White sugar, brown sugar, high-fructose corn syrup—these chemically created, highly addictive substances dramatically raise glucose levels, creating artificial energy bursts that lead to energy crashes, prompting mood swings and depression as the brain starts demanding its chemical fix. Refined sugar is as addictive as cocaine and heroin, lighting up the same pleasure centers in the brain. In the sixteenth century, the royal courts of Europe enjoyed refined sugar as a recreational drug for this very reason!

I can emphatically state that refined sugar is one of the biggest obstacles to health and beauty our country has ever encountered. The saddest part of this is that so much of our food marketed toward children is loaded with high-fructose corn syrup, and this dangerous chemical shapes the taste buds and eating patterns of an entire generation. We are now the most obese country on earth and there is no end to this in sight unless we start making better carbohydrate choices.

One of the largest beauty-killing threats posed by refined sugar is glycation, which destroys the smoothness and flexibility of the skin. When a sugar molecule bonds, or cross-links, with a lipid or protein, it creates advanced glycation end products (AGEs). These AGEs are problematic for two main reasons. First, they create ongoing inflammation in the body as they float around in the bloodstream. The immune system considers them to be foreign invaders and mounts a constant inflammatory response against them. Second, the beauty proteins collagen and elastin get destroyed when attached to these proteins. This turns beautiful, elastic, soft skin into wrinkled, leathery skin over time.

My best advice to combat glycation is to follow the guidelines of Traditional Chinese Medicine. Their key beauty strategy is to elim-

The Most Common Ways of Consuming Refined Sugar

- Regular soft drinks: 33%
  (The average American drinks
  53 *gallons* of soft drinks
  per year!)

- Sugars and candy: 16.1%
- Cakes and cookies: 9.7%
- Dairy desserts and milk: 8.6%
- Grains: 5.8%

inate cravings for refined sugars through the consumption of bitter herbs and the use of all five flavors (salty, bitter, sour, pungent, and sweet). This has a profound effect over time, adjusting our taste buds. By eating bitter herbs, fermented foods, and fresh vegetables, we give our taste buds a reset, away from the excessively sweet, which reduces our cravings for it.

Digestible Complex Carbohydrates (Polysaccharides)

Starch, glycogen, inulin, and cellulose digest more slowly because the body needs to put some work into breaking them down into mono-saccharides. This is why a bowl of steel-cut oats will give you more steady energy and keep you feeling satiated longer than a piece of fruit. Complex carbs can be found in barley, beans, brown rice, lentils, millet, oats, quinoa, and vegetables such as potatoes, squash, and sweet potatoes.

Indigestible Complex Carbohydrates (Fiber)

Cells don't source nutrients from fiber because it cannot be absorbed by the body. However, it's critical to keeping things "moving" through the digestive system, if you know what I mean. There are two types of fiber, soluble and insoluble, and we need to make sure both are in our diet.

Soluble Fiber. Soluble fiber is found inside plant cells and turns into a gel-type paste when mixed with the water in the digestive tract. This helps to soften our stool, increase the absorption of nutrients, and regulate our cholesterol levels. It keeps us feeling full for longer so we don't overeat.

Insoluble Fiber. Insoluble fiber is found in the walls of plant cells and is key to avoiding constipation. It doesn't break down in the presence of water, so it adds mass to our stool, helping things move along.

Simple carbohydrates, digestible complex carbohydrates, and indigestible complex carbohydrates are equally important to us, so it's important to make sure we incorporate all three types into our diet. Stick to carbs like organic and/or wild fruits, root vegetables, dark

---

Sad Facts About Sugar

- Added sugar alone accounts for more than 500 calories in the Standard American Diet, the caloric equivalent of ten strips of bacon every day.
- Americans consume ten times more sugar than other food additives (besides salt).
- Refined sugar has no nutritional value: zero vitamins, zero minerals, zero enzymes, zero fiber.
- Refined sugar is linked to obesity, high blood pressure, hypoglycemia, depression, headaches, fatigue, nervous tension, aching limbs, diabetes, acne, skin irritation, and stiffening of arteries.
- Processed, or refined, sugar is as addictive as cocaine.

leafy greens, raw nuts and seeds, seaweeds, and—my favorite—raw cacao. You will see and feel the difference that avoiding refined carbs makes when you start choosing nutrient-dense, beauty-enhancing unrefined carbs instead.

PROTEIN

I am a walking mass of protein, and so are you! Next to water, protein makes up the greatest portion of our body weight. The most abundant protein within us is collagen. This key protein contributes to shiny hair, smooth skin, strong nails, and healthy bones, and keeps ligaments and tendons supple. Thanks to collagen, we're able to move, bend, and stretch without pain. Another critical beauty protein, keratin, stops hair from becoming dry and brittle, nails from breaking easily, and skin from looking dull and wrinkled.

Protein helps us grow muscles and tendons, build strong tissues and ligaments, and repair cellular damage. Without protein, no organ, bone, or muscle could function properly. We wouldn't be able to make the neurotransmitters serotonin and dopamine to fuel the brain, keeping us feeling balanced and happy. We wouldn't be able to make the insulin in our pancreas, or the thyroxine secreted by our thyroid. Every single function in the body relies on protein because the cells rely on protein.

Amino Acids

When we look deeper into the structure of protein, we see it is composed of twenty-two amino acids as well as hydrogen, oxygen, carbon, nitrogen, and sometimes phosphorus and sulfur. It's the amino acids that are used by the microscopic machinery within cells as powerful building blocks for all the vital tasks they perform in the body.

Of the twenty-two amino acids that form protein, only thirteen are created by the body. The remaining nine we must take in through our food. When a food contains all nine essential amino acids, we call it a "complete protein." Several of my favorite plant-based foods meet this standard: AFA algae, almonds, amaranth, bee pollen, black beans, buckwheat, chia seeds, chickpeas, chlorella, hemp, kidney beans, marine phytoplankton, pumpkin seeds, quinoa, seaweed, and spirulina.

There is a common myth out there that you can't eat enough protein on a plant-based diet. Science has proven this to be untrue. In reality, cooked animal muscles (meats) are poor-quality protein sources. Cooking coagulates the proteins and destroys the natural enzymes. This makes the proteins harder to digest, and, even worse, turns them into inflammatory compounds within the body.

Conversely, the elastic, lightweight amino acids in uncooked plant foods are highly digestible and fully able to be utilized by the body. The most available sources of plant-based protein are almonds, bee pollen, blue-green algae, chlorella, durian, goji berries, grass (powders and the mature blades before they have flowered), green leafy vegetables (including arugula, broccoli, brussels sprouts, collards, green cabbage, kale, parsley, and spinach), hemp seeds and protein

---

The Nine Essential Amino Acids

- Histidine
- Isoleucine
- Leucine
- Lysine
- Methionine
- Phenylalanine
- Threonine
- Tryptophan
- Valine

powder, Incan berries, maca, marine phytoplankton, olives, propolis, pumpkin seeds, spirulina, sprouted grains, sprouted wild rice, and watercress.

When people say they can't possibly get enough protein without eating animal flesh, I like to point out that all the strongest, largest animals on earth feed their enormous bodies with plants—especially algae, green leaves, and plankton.

Probiotics

Scientists have discovered that our bodies are 90 percent microbial with over 100 trillion microbes living inside of us. We all have "good" and "bad" bacteria, and eating (organic) raw and fermented food is the way to tip the scale in favor of beneficial bacteria. Fermented foods produce probiotics that populate the digestive system with live enzymes and microflora. These bacteria help the body by detoxifying it, strengthening the immune system, assisting with metabolism, supporting good digestion, reducing inflammation in the gut, and manufacturing important vitamins. You can measure your health by the amount of beneficial bacteria in your body because it is a direct reflection of your inner environment.

Enzymes

Enzymes are tiny proteins found in living cells in raw foods. They act as catalysts within the body to speed up chemical reactions and aid in the digestive process by breaking down large molecules.

Digestion of food begins in the mouth. When the food reaches the stomach, it undergoes a hefty period of chemical processing due to the hydrochloric acid (HCL) there. Unfortunately, as we age our HCL naturally decreases. If we aren't proactive about counteracting this decrease by increasing our enzyme intake, we begin to accumulate undigested food materials in our intestines leading to inflammation, weight gain, bloating, skin eruptions, and overall fatigue.

PROTEIN POWDER

Protein powders are one of the most consumed supplements in the country, and yet their quality is mostly unregulated by the Food and Drug Administration (FDA). Unfortunately, this means many people seeking a quick meal replacement or a boost of protein after a workout are also drinking down lead, arsenic, mercury, cadmium, artificial flavors and colors, genetically modified organisms (GMOs), processed soy, synthetic nutrients, and toxic chemical sweeteners.

The majority of protein powders on the market are heat processed to high temperatures, which twists the proteins, halting the body from processing them as a legitimate fuel source. This means instead of providing us with easy-to-break-down amino acid–based energy to power the cells, they cause digestive problems, inflammation, and dehydration and open the door to cellular disease. Milk-based proteins like whey and casein are the favorites of many athletes, but the sad reality is that the body is not meant to process these appropriately for nourishment and over time they can end up doing us more harm than good.

Reach for a whole-food, plant-based protein powder and make sure you check the sourcing of the ingredients. I recommend Food for the Immortals Protein Drink Mix as a high-quality option. It combines bioavailable clean proteins (fermented and sprouted brown rice, pea, and amaranth) with superfoods, digestive enzymes, prebiotics, and probiotics.

I recommend consuming plant enzymes, as they remain alive and working within the wide pH range of the stomach and intestines. They are effective in both areas to break up incoming food, destroy compacted food residue, and keep digestion flowing. Enzymes from animal sources are eventually killed by the low pH of the stomach and therefore do not travel onto the intestines to aid in digestion there, making them a less viable choice.

GREEN VEGETABLES, FRUITS, NUTS, SEEDS, SPROUTS, AND SEA VEGETABLES

GREEN VEGETABLES

Green (especially leafy) vegetables are probably one of the most important groups of foods. There's practically no system within the body that won't benefit from them. They provide fiber and alkalinity to keep us clean on the inside, which in turn keeps us glowing on the outside.

Green veggies have many calming, anti-stress properties and are some of the best sources of minerals, fiber, silica (beauty bomb!), and chlorophyll. Chlorophyll is one of nature's greatest healers and can neutralize bad breath and body odor almost instantly. All these properties are absolutely essential to maintain a youthful and radiant complexion.

Any and all green leafy vegetables are great for you. Think: *Neutralize, deodorize, and detoxify!* Try to eat them raw to reap the maximum benefits, and of course wild, homegrown, and/or organic whenever possible. The following are some of my favorites.

Kale has finally hit the big time. It is one of the best sources in all of nature of the important blood coagulant vitamin K_1. Kale has also been shown to lower the harmful type of cholesterol and decrease the body's absorption of bad fat and oil. Plus, it has antioxidants—including a high ORAC (oxygen radical absorbance capacity) score on a par with the almighty blueberry!

Parsley has always been one of my favorite vegetables. Even as a child, I used to eat the parsley garnish on my plate instead of throwing it away. I've always loved how concentrated parsley is. You do not have to eat much to get the alkaline power of this special vegetable. It is the best source of chlorophyll and carotenoids of any land plant, and a unique thing about parsley is its high iron content (5 to 8 milligrams per 100 grams).

Okay, **radishes** aren't always green, but they are an incredible health and beauty food! They are high in fiber, support digestion, have excellent antibacterial and anti-inflammatory properties, aid in detoxification, and contain isothiocyanates, which buffer the body against potential carcinogens. Full of essential fatty acids, minerals, and vitamins (especially vitamin C), radishes protect your glowing, hydrated skin from environmental damage.

Burdock root is one of the classic "magical herbs" and has been used in traditional Ayurveda for thousands of years to purify the blood and alleviate skin conditions, such as infections, rashes, and eczema. It's super concentrated in all the beauty vitamins and minerals, including B_1, B_2, B_3, C, iron, silicon, manganese, and zinc, and it's a neutrally pH balanced root, whereas most roots are acidic. The high mineral content, supported with its brilliant white inner flesh, also makes it an excellent beautifier of the teeth!

Some other awesome green vegetable choices include

- Artichokes
- Arugula
- Asparagus
- Beet greens
- Bell peppers
- Cabbage
- Celery
- Chard
- Collards
- Leeks
- Romaine lettuce
- Spinach
- Watercress

FRUITS

Fruits are the most enchanting (and egotistical!) of all food groups. Fruits show us everything and display their beauty! In addition to their fair share of amino acids (and sometimes essential fatty acids), fruits are excellent sources of many nutrients, including color pigment antioxidants, water, potassium, dietary fiber, vitamin C, and folate. The combination of powerful flavonoids, antioxidants, minerals, vitamins, phytochemicals, and countless micro- and macronutrients make them a smart part of your health and beauty regimen. Plus, they are broken down and absorbed quickly by the body, so they are a great source of quick energy, supporting weight loss by providing ample stamina and nearly every nutrient your body needs without adding any unnecessary fats.

A fruit is an edible product of a plant that contains the seeds for reproduction. This is why we want to be sure that we eat only fruits with seeds—otherwise we will become *seedless*. Got it? For the best bang for your beauty buck, choose fruits that are hydrating, low-glycemic, alkaline, and as highly rated on the ORAC scale as possible. Based on the minerals they contain, some fruits are classified as alkaline, some neutral, and some acidic—they vary a great deal. Alkaline fruits are the best ever, but it is important to remember that even the most acidic fruits are still not nearly as acidic as grains, nuts, or meat over the long term.

As with green vegetables, try to eat your fruits raw, wild, home-grown, and/or organic whenever possible. The following are some of my favorites.

All **berries** are just so *good* for you on so many different levels. Berries are some of the most effective disease-fighting foods available and have some of the highest measured ORAC levels. They contain plenty of fiber, catechins (a flavonoid compound), gallic acid (an antioxidant that has been shown to inhibit cancerous cell proliferation), ellagic acid (a phenolic compound that is also a potent anticarcinogen), and anthocyanins (the color pigments in berries that do all kinds of wonderful things, including improve memory, keep skin firm, support overall healthy aging, and decrease the risk of developing certain cancers). I'd say incorporating berries into your diet should be at the top of your list. I'm in Canada right now, writing this book, and I just harvested all our cherries and berries. I have been eating copious amounts of cherries, raspberries, and super beautifying seabuckthorn berries all day long!

Cantaloupe is such an interesting melon. It contains a remarkable diversity of nutrients, including huge amounts of vitamin C and about thirty times more carotenoids than oranges. It ranks high in B vitamins (including folate) as well as vitamin K, potassium, magnesium, and fiber. It also contains an impressive amount of omega-3, in the form of alpha-linolenic acid (stacking the odds in your favor for the best skin ever), and possesses the flavonoid luteolin, the antioxidant organic acids ferulic and caffeic, and the anti-inflammatory cucurbitacins B and E. Here's what all this means: strengthened immune system; improved heart health; reduced stress; prevented hair loss;

THE DIRTY DOZEN

It is my recommendation that you eat as many fruits and vegetables as you can each day since they pack a tremendous beauty punch and they work synergistically to give you the most beautiful skin, hair, nails, and teeth. However, toxic chemicals are sprayed on these foods when they are conventionally grown, and with each bite of chemical-laden produce, you add to the toxic load on your body. With beauty, the inside is as important as the outside. It is particularly important to keep your liver and kidneys working at optimal function.

Every year the Environmental Working Group compiles a list of 48 of the most contaminated fruits and vegetables on the market, with the top 12 on that list called the "Dirty Dozen." The following list is based on the most recent analysis of over 36,000 produce samples taken by the United States Department of Agriculture (USDA) and the FDA. I recommend that when you eat these foods, you choose to either grow them yourself or buy organic.

1. Apples
2. Celery
3. Cherries
4. Cucumbers
5. Grapes
6. Nectarines
7. Peaches
8. Pears
9. Spinach
10. Strawberries
11. Sweet bell peppers
12. Tomatoes

soft, conditioned hair; clear, bright eyes; weight loss; and a whole lot of hydration, regeneration, and rejuvenation.

Lemons, oranges, limes—citrus fruits aid the body by flushing out kidney and liver toxins via improved hydration, jump-starting the digestive tract with citric acid, and supporting healing with their extraordinary content of vitamin C. To increase detoxification, start each morning with a warm glass of lemon water.

Pineapple is perhaps most famous for its tremendous bromelain and vitamin C content. The dream team combination of this enzyme and water-soluble vitamin is great for healthy, shiny hair; the repair and prevention of fine lines; clear, soft, blemish-free skin; and healthy cell regeneration. This bromeliad has been used for thousands of years in South America as a natural anti-inflammatory and throat/vocal relaxant and rejuvenator. Pineapple is from the Amazon basin originally and, for me, connects naturally to the far-seeing third eye of Amazonian shamans—pineapple dissolves pineal gland calcification.

Other great fruit choices for beauty include
- Apples
- Avocados
- Cherries
- Cucumbers
- Figs
- Grapefruits
- Grapes (varieties with seeds)
- Kiwi
- Okra
- Olives
- Papaya
- Pears
- Pomegranates
- Tangerines

Acid–Alkaline Balance

Achieving optimal nutritional balance boils down to understanding and continually working to maintain a proper acidic to alkaline range in your diet. The measurement of acidity or alkalinity is often referred to as pH (potential hydrogen). The pH scale ranges from totally acidic at 0.0 to totally alkaline at 14.0, with 7.0 being neutral. The body generally uses electrolytes (calcium, lithium, magnesium, phosphorus, potassium, and sodium) to control pH levels. An ideal blood pH is from 7.35 to 7.40, though some tissues in the body are more acidic, such as the muscles and skin, which optimally come in at 6.8. So when the pH measurements of tissues are added together and averaged, the number should be around 7.0. However, people who predominantly survive on the Standard American Diet are unbalanced and acidic, with an overall pH as low as 6.2 (and sometimes even lower).

Acidity tends to be the underlying cause of all ailments that spoil beauty. Acidity creates inflammation, puffiness, asymmetry, and contraction of the tissues. The only way to correct this imbalance is to eat a ratio of foods that are more alkaline than acidic and to get in the habit of drinking more high-quality spring water. But it's not as simple as avoiding acidic foods, because we need both alkali- and acid-forming foods to be healthy and in balance. Minerals run 95 percent of the body's activities, so human biochemistry is completely dependent on varied mineral content, a primary determinant of the acidity of a food. Foods rich in alkaline minerals (calcium, iron, magnesium, manganese, silicon, and sodium) support alkalinity in the body. Foods rich in acidic minerals (iodine, nitrogen, phosphorous, and sulfur) promote acidity in the body. Preliminary research has shown that deep breathing can promote alkalinity as well.

Alkalinizing fruits: blackberries, citrus fruits (grapefruits, lemons, limes, oranges, etc.), cranberries, figs, grapes (varieties with seeds), hot chilies, kiwi, okra, olives, papaya, passion fruit, pineapple, pomegranates, raspberries

Neutral fruits: apples, apricots, bell peppers, blueberries, cucumbers, guava, jackfruit, lychee, mango, mangosteen, melons, noni, peaches, pumpkin, strawberries, tomatoes

Acid-balancing fruits: avocados, bananas, cacao, dates, dried fruits (except figs), durians, grapes (seedless varieties), mulberries, plums, prunes

NUTS AND SEEDS

Nuts and seeds are nutrient dense. They provide vitamins, minerals, natural enzymes, and quick energy without unhealthy fat or empty calories. Adding them into and/or sprinkling them onto your meals will often ensure that you fill in nutritional gaps—and they are awesome supporters of collagen production! Always try to eat raw, organic (and preferably soaked—see page 40) nuts and seeds to reap maximum benefits and to avoid unhealthy toxins, like synthetic fertilizers and pesticides.

Nuts

Besides being packed with protein, nuts provide monounsaturated and polyunsaturated fats, omega-3 fatty acids, fiber, vitamin E, L-arginine, and more. They can lower bad cholesterol, support a healthy heart, and help control free radicals. Plus, they are an easy snack that will fill you up, reduce cravings, curtail inflammation, promote cell regeneration, and keep your skin glowing. A word to the wise: Eat nuts! But don't eat too many or you may go nuts (and gain weight . . . and feel bloated).

Here are some of the most "nut"-worthy choices:

Almonds may be one of the most perfect foods for your skin. Their protein content supports collagen production, and their high concentrations of vitamins B_1, B_5, B_6, and E, calcium, copper, zinc, and monounsaturated fats are all super skin-friendly too. Stress is a killer for skin health, so the magnesium content that bolsters your nervous system will benefit your epidermis as well.

Walnuts contain a number of neuroprotective compounds, including vitamin E, folate, melatonin, omega-3 fatty acids, and antioxidants.

How to Soak Nuts and Seeds

Add 1 teaspoon Himalayan or Celtic sea salt along with your organic nuts or seeds into a glass bowl. Pour warm water over the nuts or seeds until your ratio of water to nuts or seeds is roughly two to one. Ideally you want to soak them overnight or for about seven hours. (Adding salt is important because it helps reduce the enzyme inhibitors that make nuts and seeds so hard to digest.)

They are exceptional for internal cleansing, immune system support, brain health (don't they look just like little brains, after all?), and candida growth deterrence. They are proficient anti-agers for skin and hair, moisturizing and hydrating cells, brightening and lightening dark circles under the eyes, and making hair longer, stronger, and shinier.

Chestnuts are much lower in fat and calories than most other nuts, but they are one of the highest in dietary fiber and are impressively high in protein and water content. Chestnuts have a whopping 30 percent of the recommended dietary allowance of vitamin C and are a great source of B vitamins, copper, magnesium, and iron. They increase bone mineral density, prevent the breakdown of collagen, keep the immune system healthy and strong, and improve cognitive function.

Seeds

Like nuts, seeds are a vital part of a healthy, beautifying diet. They are high in fiber, monounsaturated fats, and vitamin E, and they are a great source of protein, minerals, zinc, and many other life- and beauty-enhancing nutrients. Avoid irradiated seeds, and try to eat them in only a raw, organic state. Some of my favorites are cashews, pumpkin seeds, chia seeds, and hemp seeds. Other awesome choices are sunflower seeds, sesame seeds, and coconuts, which are so special, they are at the top of my list and are discussed in great length in the "Superfoods and Superherbs" chapter (page 49).

In case you are new to adding nuts and seeds into your diet, be sure to soak them in pure water overnight, then dehydrate them to a crisp before eating, whenever possible. Soaking nuts and seeds in water tends to make them more alkaline and digestible by deactivating phytic acid and enzyme inhibitors.

SPROUTS

You will hear me say this over and over again: *Plant a garden*. If you do not have access to a patch of land for a garden, start a sprout garden in your kitchen. This is something everyone can do, and the rewards will be huge. Every plant-based food starts as a sprout, so there are many, many, many to choose from, including clover sprouts, broccoli sprouts, sunflower sprouts, sprouted grasses (e.g., wheatgrass, kamut, or barley), mung bean sprouts, rye sprouts, hemp seed sprouts, chia sprouts, radish sprouts, fenugreek sprouts, alfalfa sprouts, coconut sprouts, and more. These are all super concentrated little nutrition powerhouses.

Sprouts are full of proteolytic enzymes, which help the body digest proteins and carbohydrates and absorb nutrients. As you age, it gets harder for your body to produce these on its own, so adding spouts into your diet is an excellent way to pick up the slack. Also, sprouts are an impressive source of fiber, minerals, protein, B vitamins, iron, magnesium, phosphorous, and potassium.

Broccoli sprouts are one of my all-time favorite sprouts. They pack sulforaphane, which in scientific studies has been shown to reduce

How to Sprout Seeds

Make sure you sprout from only organic, non-GMO, raw seeds that have not been pasteurized or irradiated. Fill a clean mason jar up to one-quarter full with seeds. Top the jar with fresh spring water, then cover the jar with a mesh sprouting screen. Soak the seeds overnight at room temperature. Be sure to keep the sprouting jar away from light or cover with a towel. The soak time should be at least five hours for small seeds and up to twelve hours for large seeds and grains. In the morning, drain the jar and rinse the seeds. Place the jar on its side for a few hours so air can circulate and the rinse water can continue to drain off. Repeat this entire process three times a day for three days or until the seeds sprout. When you start seeing little green leaves develop, they are ready to eat! Sunflower sprouts are an exception; they need to be sprouted in a tray of potting soil.

breast cancer cell clusters and keep *Helicobacter pylori*—nasty bacteria associated with the proliferation of cancer—at bay. A review of sprouts in human nutrition found the following:

> Based on the data of the literature it can be stated that the original composition of the seeds essentially changes during germination. The quantity of the protein fractions changes, the proportion of the nitrogen containing fractions shifts toward the smaller protein fractions, oligopeptides and free amino acids. Beyond this changes the quantity of the amino acids (some of them increase, others decrease or do not alter) during germination, and nonprotein amino acids also are produced. In consequence of these changes, the biological value of the sprout protein increases, and greater digestibility was established in animal experiments. The composition of the triglycerides also changes, owing to hydrolysis, free fatty acids originate, [which] can be considered as a certain kind of predigestion. Generally, the ratio of the saturated fatty acids increases compared

to unsaturated fatty acids, and the ratio within the unsaturated fatty acids shifts to the essential linoleic acid. The quantity of the antinutritive materials decreases, and the utilization of the macro and micro elements is increased owing to germination. Furthermore the sprouts contain many such materials (sulphoraphane, sulphoraphene, isothiocyanates, gluco-sinolates, enzymes, antioxidants, vitamins) that are proved to be effective in the prevention of cancer, or in the therapy against cancer.[*]

SEA VEGETABLES AND ALGAE

Rich in life-giving nutrients drawn from the ocean and the sun, sea vegetables—also known as seaweeds—help remove heavy metals, detoxify the body, provide numerous trace minerals, nourish with polysaccharides (essential sugars), regulate cholesterol, and decrease the risk of cancer. Seaweeds benefit the entire body but are especially excellent for the thyroid (since they're high in iodine), the immune system, the adrenals, and hormone function. They cleanse, tone, and moisturize skin; uplift the mood; and prevent premature pigmentation.

Arame, bladderwrack, dulse, hijiki, kelp, nori, sea lettuce, and sea palm are some powerful seaweeds that can easily be incorporated into your diet. I also recommend experimenting with and finding the superfood complete protein algae that agree with you: AFA (aphani-zomenon flos-aquae) blue-green algae, chlorella, marine phytoplankton, and spirulina. I typically recommend chlorella the most. Chlorella is an edible microalgae that has the highest chlorophyll content of any food in the world, at 10 percent chlorophyll by dry matter weight—that is about fifty times higher in chlorophyll than quality green vegetables. This makes chlorella one of the most powerful detoxifying substances known. Blue-green algae such as spirulina and AFA are others I

---

[*] M. Márton, Zs. Mándoki, Zs. Csapó-Kiss, and J. Csapó, "The Role of Sprouts in Human Nutrition: A Review," *Alimentaria* 3 (2010): 81–117, http://www.isga-sprouts.org/wp -content/uploads/2014/03/TheRoleofSproutsinHumanNutrition-MelyndaMarton.pdf.

recommend that are heavily utilized by millions of people. They both contain the blue pigment phycocyanin; this super rare blue pigment possesses numerous benefits including joint protection, more stem cell production, neurotransmitter formation, and acting to block the COX-2 and lipoxygenase enzymes, thus delivering anti-inflammatory effects. Marine phytoplankton are also promising, as certain varieties, such as *Nannochloropsis gaditana*, contain the fish oil DHA (docosahexaenoic acid) in a plant-based form with numerous antioxidant carotenoids and absorption-enhancing phospholipids.

THE AYURVEDIC APPROACH TO A BALANCED DIET

Eating for Your Dosha

There is a "best" way to eat according to Ayurveda, and it relates to your unique body type based on your dominant *doshas,* or body energies. Everyone has three doshas within them: *kapha, pitta,* and *vata.* The doshas relate to the five elements: space, air, fire, water, and earth. Usually one or two doshas are dominant in your body, determining your personality, your general likes and dislikes, and how you metabolize your food. Discovering your dominant dosha or doshas and then learning what corresponding foods are ideal for you is one of the most effective ways to nourish your body. It can save you a lot of time and energy trying to slim down your waistline and repair damaged skin. Please visit www.beautydietbook.com to discover which dosha(s) you are!

Kapha: A combination of water and earth elements, kaphas are people who tend to have strong immune systems and more relaxed dispositions. They need to eat less food than the other doshas as their bodies like to hold on to weight. Kaphas have enviable skin when they are in balance, as it's naturally hydrated. Dry brushing is great for kaphas. (See "Dry Brushing," page 130.)

Kapha body types need to reduce sweet, heavy, and wet foods and consume mostly hot and dry foods. Their digestive fire can be low and should be stoked with herbs and spices to keep their metabolisms up. They do better with hot drinks than with cold, and they should reduce their oil intake and use dairy sparingly, as they are prone to phlegm. Vigorous and regular exercise is very helpful for this body type to boost metabolism and avoid overall body stagnation. Kapha-balancing foods include apple cider vinegar, beets, carrots, cilantro, dried fruit, ginger, mustard greens, peppers, and radishes.

Pitta: The energy of fire burns bright with pittas, who have dynamic metabolic systems and a warm constitution. People of this short-tempered dosha can usually eat a large amount of food with little weight gain. They tend to be slim because they burn calories fast and don't need as much exercise as kaphas. They are prone to oily skin issues like rashes and acne and have sensitive skin, which means commercial cosmetics can wreak havoc on their faces and cause severe skin reactions.

Pittas must emphasize cooling things down. Eating cooling foods and enjoying cold drinks are easy ways to balance pittas. Good-quality fats are great for this dosha, as reactions to processed, rancid fats can lead to massive acne outbreaks.

Pitta-balancing foods include asparagus, celery, coconut oil, fresh fruits (avocados, cucumbers, grapes, melons, papaya, pineapple), ghee, and olive oil.

Vata: A light, dry dosha associated with the elements of wind and space, vatas are the dosha of motion and the circulatory system. They tend to have light frames and thin builds. Vatas are balanced best by stability and routine, and when they become imbalanced can feel very unstable. Vatas are most susceptible to dry skin and therefore must use topical oils regularly and drink lots of water. If they live in a windy environment, they must protect their skin. A common beauty killer for vatas is lack of sleep or poor-quality sleep. Their bedtime routine should include a warming tea, a relaxing environment, and a moisturizing ritual.

Vatas do not do well on a raw food diet, so warm foods, like soup, are ideal for their constitution. Coffee aggravates this dosha more than the others; ginger tea is a great alternative. Having a set meal plan may feel counterintuitive for a vata, but eating on a consistent schedule will work physical wonders for this dosha. They must avoid yo-yo dieting and the extremes of fasting and bingeing.

Vata-balancing foods include avocados, bananas, beets, coconut, ghee, mango, olives, squash, sweet potato, and watercress.

CONCLUSION

Fats, carbohydrates, and proteins form the necessary elements of the human diet. This means that each of these food classes must be present in some significant percentage in the diet. The percentage for each class varies from person to person, depending on their metabolic type, current state of digestion, health history, health goals, etc. Regardless of which of these macronutrients you feel is most important, the truth is, they *all* are. Don't make the mistake of starving your body of any of these three key components in an attempt to achieve beaming beauty and overall wellness. Eat plenty of healthy plant-based fats, choose high-fiber carbs, and get adequate protein. Listen to your body's cues, and maintain balanced levels of each, depending on your specific needs.

Nothing is as indicative of inner health, youthful vigor, and external beauty as a strong, energized person with glowing skin and clear, sparkling eyes! In order to have soft cheeks and silky, radiant skin, you must choose a lifestyle that rises above food dogma and is actually favorable to skin beauty. The skin is always the last organ to be nourished, because it is the farthest away from the digestive organs— and that's also why it is important to nourish the skin naturally from the outside in with coconut oil, cacao butter, seabuckthorn oil, and/ or olive oil. Care of the skin runs deep and requires diligence and discipline; yet skin care begins with internal cleanliness and properly balanced plant-based food choices.

Superfoods
and Superherbs
The Building Blocks of Beauty

SUPERFOODS

Superfoods are both food and medicine. They are the most powerful, concentrated, nutrient-dense foods on earth, giving us the biggest nutritional bang for our buck. I believe that by incorporating superfoods into your diet regularly you can awaken your potential to experience radiant health and enjoy youthful, glowing skin and strong, thick hair and nails. These foods will help you look and feel the *best ever* in your body.

The science of superfoods is straightforward. Maximizing the body's intake of specific plants provides it with good, whole sources of hormone-free, pesticide-free, non-GMO minerals, vitamins, antioxidants, fats and oils, amino acids, glyconutrients, enzymes, coenzymes, and polysaccharides. By adding in foods like cacao, coconut, goji, and maca, you give your body a tremendous advantage for cell repair, free-radical elimination, hormone balancing, and better sleep, which results in a beautiful, glowing exterior.

Today, because we live in a radiation-filled, mineral-depleted, chemical-laden world, plant consumption needs to go beyond just the regular organic vegetables in order to keep us detoxified and fueled properly. While organic veggies, fruits, nuts, seeds, sprouts, and sea vegetables are important parts of an overall beauty diet, these foods do not even come close to the nutritional density of superfoods, so it's important that *these too* be part of a well-rounded food plan.

Eating superfoods guarantees the body the nutrients it needs to radiate inner health. They are an extremely satisfying, easy, and delicious way to get in all the key beauty nutrients while increasing your life force and extending your life span. They fuel you on a level that ordinary foods, even organic foods, simply can't.

When you look deep into their structural components, superfoods flaunt more than a dozen unique characteristics and provide you with dense, complex nutrition to nourish you down to your cellular matrix. Superfoods have a long history of use in Ayurveda and Chinese tonic herbalism. Why? Because they work.

One purpose of this book is to provide simple tips that will upgrade what you are already doing. If you currently drink sodas, you can upgrade your nutritional operating system by replacing 8 ounces of soda a day with a glass of goji tea or spring water. If you decide to eat a salad, upgrade it to superfood status by adding spirulina or chlorella to it. Get rid of your white processed salt and start sprinkling Icelandic sea salt on your food. Throw out the fake pasteurized honey in the squeeze bottle and start consuming raw organic honey. By taking these small steps, you begin to stack the odds in your favor to experience the best health ever—every day of your life—activating your ability to be infinitely beautiful.

Food is not just *a* factor that affects us, it is *the* primary factor that affects us. Understanding this makes it easier to choose foods that add to your health and beauty, rather than defaulting into inflammatory foods and foods we're allergic to. Your inner radiance and magnetism are fueled by the foods you eat and the liquids you drink. Many lifestyle factors affect beauty, including exercise, sleep, and the amount of stress in your life, but nutrition is the cornerstone of beauty.

Nature provides the best raw materials to create beauty from the inside out. Superfruits (such as goji berries and acai), beautify you; green foods, such as spirulina and aloe vera keep your system clean on the inside with fiber and balanced alkalinity; they also mineralize you to create healthy bones, skin, hair, and nails; high-quality, fresh fats and oils (such as avocados, olives, and young coconut) restore elasticity to your tissues and give you a youthful appearance. These foods add shine to your eyes, glow to your hair, energy to your day, and strength to your body. You will look better, feel better, and function better. And *that* is beautiful.

Let's dig in to the twelve most potent superfoods to fuel your internal and external appearance so you can shine and glow like the radiant being you are. These foods are a must for any beauty regimen.

The Top Twelve Superfoods for Beauty

- Acai
- Aloe vera
- Avocado
- Cacao
- Coconut oil
- Goji berries
- Hemp seeds and seed oil
- Honey
- Maca
- Olive oil
- Pumpkin seeds and seed oil
- Spirulina

Warning: These foods will cause you to have the most beautiful day ever!

ACAI

The legendary acai berry is really a date that grows on a tropical palm tree. Acai made its grand entrance into the West in the early 1990s, though tribes in the Amazon jungle have been consuming it for thousands of years. Traditionally, it has been celebrated for its ability to boost the immune system, increase energy, fight infections, support a healthy heart, and increase sex drive. Tribal shamans have also used it as an antibiotic and treatment for parasitic conditions like schistosomiasis, ulcers, diarrhea, and bleeding disorders.

But acai is not just helpful during times of illness; it is also a highly coveted energy and beauty tonic. When Western surfers were introduced to the energy-enhancing and "natural Viagra" effects of acai and brought it north, it exploded onto the health food scene. By the aughts, acai was exported from Brazil all over the world. Since it is best eaten fresh, the berries are usually handpicked and immediately pulped, flash-pasteurized, and frozen or freeze-dried. Acai can now be found in most supermarkets all over the world as a powder, as a refrigerated juice, or in the frozen foods section. It can be blended into smoothies, made into teas, or applied directly to the skin and hair.

Low in sugar and high in all the good stuff, acai berries are some of the most nutritious and delicious little fruits you will ever find. It is an excellent source of fiber, protein, iron, vitamin A, vitamin E, and calcium. The berries have over-the-top levels of anthocyanins (estimated to be ten to thirty times higher than those of red wine!) and are also rich in plant sterols. These powerful antioxidants support healthy cholesterol levels and robust blood composition and circulation. Acai has mega amounts of essential fatty acids too (omega-3, omega-6, and omega-9), which are well known for keeping your cells saturated with enough nutrients and hydration to support super healthy skin and hair. Acai helps revive tired, damaged skin cells, restore moisture, relieve the inflammatory effects of acne, protect your skin from the harmful and premature aging effects of environmental toxins and air pollution by helping to smooth fine lines and hyperpigmentation, and restore an overall vibrant complexion for more youthful-looking skin.

To support strong, thick, soft locks, try adding acai to a hair rinse. (You may want to avoid applying this topically if you have chemically treated or naturally blond hair, as it will stain through several washes.)

For soft, plump lips, make a deliciously nourishing and naturally tinted lip balm:

Acai Lip Balm

1 tablespoon beeswax

1 tablespoon mango butter

1 tablespoon coconut oil

Acai berry powder

Combine all the ingredients well, adding acai berry powder until you achieve your desired richness of color.

ALOE VERA

Aloe is hands down nature's best emollient. Being high in methylsulfonylmethane (MSM), it has the ability to heal sunburns and other burns quickly. It's also loaded with enzymes, particularly bradykinase, which is an inflammation fighter and skin soother. There have been numerous reports showing the positive role aloe plays in healing psoriasis, dermatitis, and burn injuries.

Aloe vera makes the skin more elastic and smooth, and helps to maintain the skin's microbiome (community of healthy bacteria) without destroying beneficial skin bacteria, unlike harsh soaps and petroleum-based moisturizers. Its power to enhance collagen and elastin, along with its ability to soothe, hydrate, and nourish, makes aloe vera the number one topical superfood for skin regeneration and repair.

Raw aloe gel is made up mostly of water and long-chain sugars (polysaccharides), and it contains numerous exotic nutrients including anthraquinones (laxatives), gibberellins (plant hormones that speed healing), salicylic acid (aspirin compound), anti-inflammatory sterols, and choline (protects the liver and brain), among many others. Raw aloe also contains minerals, like calcium and magnesium, as well as trace minerals, such as manganese, chromium, and copper, all of which promote radiant beauty. It is a fantastic source of zinc too, an element that keeps the immune system strong and is a key component for hormone receptors, which contribute to a balanced mood and appearance.

Did you know that aloe is just as nourishing to your hair and dry scalp as it is to your skin? Its moisturizing properties keep hair strong and healthy while its antibacterial and antifungal properties help to eliminate dandruff and the itching associated with it.

Walking down cosmetics and skin care aisles, you may see aloe sap, aloe juice, or other aloe vera derivatives listed on shampoos, makeup, sunscreens, shaving creams, and moisturizers. Unfortunately, these may be chock-full of numerous chemicals of dubious safety. Instead of buying more aloe vera products, try filleting a real aloe leaf and applying the fresh aloe gel directly to your body and see how powerful it really is.

The miraculous effects of aloe vera aren't just skin-deep. Consuming aloe vera gel heals the intestinal lining, boosts the immune system, enhances gut flora, and improves the body's ability to absorb nutrients and deliver them to the skin, all of which are essential for beauty. Aloe vera is a demulcent, meaning it relieves irritation and inflammation, and in today's world, it is critical to get these types of foods into our diet. A broken digestive system wreaks havoc on our health. Plus, the gel is anti-inflammatory and can help eliminate puffy eyes, bloating, and constipation.

Aloe vera is not a tonic and therefore should be used only occasionally, not every day, especially when using it internally. It has a very strong mechanism of action, so once or twice a week topically or internally is all you need. It is also very bitter, so I recommend mixing it with fruits or vegetables to mask the flavor.

How to Prepare Fresh Aloe Vera to Use Topically

If you are able to find a freshly sliced aloe leaf, cut off the tip, then slice carefully between the skin and the gel on both sides of the leaf, removing the skin entirely and leaving only the gel. Cut the large gel portion into palm-length pieces. Apply the gel generously to the face, being careful not to touch your eyes. Leave the gel on your face for thirty to forty minutes for maximum benefit. Use any leftover pieces in a smoothie or refrigerate.

Super Skin Elixir

This elixir combines hydrating aloe vera and coconut water, alkalizing green powder, ginger for circulation, fulvic acid for detoxification, and MSM for healthy connective tissue—all in one super amazing beverage for beautiful skin! It also contains a healthy dose of raspberries. A comparative study has shown that raspberries contain more than twenty substances that prevent tissues from aging.

8 ounces coconut water

4-inch piece fresh aloe vera, skin removed

1 orange, peeled and seeded

1 cup fresh raspberries

1 to 3 teaspoons green powder of your choice

½-inch piece fresh ginger root

2 squirts fulvic acid

1 teaspoon MSM powder

Stevia or raw organic honey to taste

Blend all the ingredients together in a high-speed blender and enjoy!

AVOCADO

The avocado is by far one of the most interesting and powerful superfoods on our beloved earth. I love it so much I've taken it as my middle name! My affinity and deep appreciation for this exqui-site fruit came out of necessity. Decades ago, when I was in my early twenties and broke while striking it out on my own in California, in order to feed myself I would forage for wild food. Being a strict vegan, I lived on a diet of mainly fruits, vegetables, and wild foods, like wild lettuce, rosemary, mustards, olives, white sapotes, lemonade berries, and whatever else was growing in my neighborhood. Avocados were my main source of calories and nourishment then and for a long time afterward. I estimate that in the course of my lifetime I have eaten over twenty thousand avocados, and counting!

With super high levels of phytosterols, carotenoids, flavonoids, and polyhydroxylated fatty alcohols, avocados are loaded with phytonu-trients that fight free radicals. They are also an excellent source of pantothenic acid, vitamins B_6, C, E, and K, potassium, copper, folate, and dietary fiber. They are one of the few fruits that provide an excellent source of polyunsaturated and monounsaturated fats too—the good kind, especially oleic acid. Plus, they act as nutrient "boosters," helping the body absorb more fat-soluble nutrients—such as lutein and alpha- and beta-carotene—from the foods eaten with them.

Polyunsaturated fats are good for the brain, muscles, and nerves, and (one more bonus) they protect the skin from the effects of sun damage. Monounsaturated fats—along with the avocado's impressively high levels of vitamins C and E—lubricate the joints and facilitate tissue hydration throughout the intestines, keeping the entire body supple. The avocado's eye protectors lutein and zeaxanthin help you remain bright-eyed and bushy-tailed. Also, the avocado's beta-carotene and lycopene have been connected to improving overall skin health and tone since they support strong cell membranes and shield skin from premature aging and wrinkles.

In addition to keeping things running smoothly on the inside, avocados naturally enhance outward beauty. To maximize the effects of this fascinating fruit, mash the raw pulp and apply it as a face mask to rehydrate dry tissues. Use it as a cooling remedy for sunburn and/or skin irritations, like psoriasis. Massage it directly into your scalp to condition dry, brittle hair and to encourage an increase of healthy hair growth.

I could go on all day about avocados! I guarantee that making them a regular part of your diet will ensure you look as radiant as you will feel after eating them!

CACAO

Chocolate is the *best superfood ever.* I love chocolate so much that I bought a farm in Hawaii and grow chocolate trees (cacao trees).

The raw cacao bean (the source of all chocolate) is what I consider

Buyer Beware

It's essential to look for cacao marked "jungle grown," the reason being that thousands of jungles around the world have been mowed down by huge corporations, sprayed with toxic chemicals to kill everything on the land, and then planted with a lab-created, hybridized, GMO version of cacao plants called CCN-51. The CCN-51 plants have almost no nutritional value, are high in phytic acid, which blocks the absorption of minerals in your body, and are sold as organic even though they are grown on land that has been poisoned with dangerous chemicals.

High-integrity companies like longevitywarehouse.com sell jungle-grown, organic, heirloom cacao products.

to be one of nature's most outstanding beauty superfoods due to its abundant mineral and trace mineral content. Just like the avocado, cacao can be eaten or applied topically, and you receive equal benefits either way.

Cacao contains protein, vitamins A and C, riboflavin, thiamine, calcium, potassium, magnesium, bioavailable iron, chromium, manganese, zinc, copper, omega-6 fatty acids, sulfur, and phosphorus. It is loaded with antioxidants that protect and repair your skin from premature aging. The oil in the cacao seed helps to improve and rejuvenate your skin's condition and appearance because it's a potent anti-inflammatory. The polyphenols in cacao also help to create healthy gut bacteria, which aid digestion. All of this assists the flow of blood throughout your body, which promotes cellular healing and increases hydration, leading to youthful, radiant skin.

Do you reach for chocolate when you're feeling stressed out or you've had a long day and just want to relax? (See page 282 for tasty Fruit and Nut Super Chocolate Cups.) There's actually a scientific reason why your body craves chocolate at these times. Cacao contains anandamide, sometimes referred to as the "bliss molecule," which hits your cannabinoid receptors like a warm hug, making you feel happier while also increasing neurogenesis, the formation of nerve cells in the brain.

COCONUT OIL

Thin is in, but saturated fat is where it's at!

As I mentioned in the previous chapter, for many years there was a campaign against saturated fat, spearheaded by US government agencies that claimed that saturated fat caused arteries to clog up. In reality, arterial damage caused by industrial seed oils (such as corn oil, safflower oil, and cottonseed oil) and overconsumption of refined carbohydrates caused this problem. Thankfully, the clarification of this point meant coconut oil went back on the "good foods" list, which was the best news ever, because it's so beautifying, both internally and externally, it would be a shame for anyone to go without it.

When I'm not traveling, I live at my agricultural center in Hawaii. I've had the chance to grow coconuts on my property and experience firsthand how this amazing tree can be used in so many life-affirming ways. I've come to develop what I would consider a deep, personal connection with the coconut. At my house, I set up a coconut cutting station, and there is nothing better than going out there in the morning with a big machete and cracking into a coconut, freshly harvested from one of the trees. It took me a while to get the hang of it, but now I can get the water out in a few chops and the meat out in a few more.

It seems counterintuitive to eat fat to lose weight, right? It's the opposite of what we were taught when growing up. Of course this lesson does apply to some fats. For example, the high-calorie, long-chain saturated fats found in animal and dairy products are hard to digest and clog up our system. But coconut oil is different. It's composed of approximately 90 percent medium-chain saturated fats, which the body can metabolize efficiently. It has fewer calories by weight than any other fat source and provides us with quick, usable energy. Plus, it has the bonus of switching on our metabolism to help us lose weight.

Raw saturated fat is an important building block of each cell in the human body. The skin and subcutaneous levels under the skin, as well as the membranes around each cell in the body, contain saturated fat. When you consume a bioavailable saturated fat source, like coconut oil, you nourish your cells. They then function at their best, which boosts your immune system, your thyroid, your digestion, and your absorption of fat-soluble vitamins, minerals like calcium and magnesium, phospholipids like choline and lecithin, and moisturizing fatty acids like omega-3s. All of these factors contribute to shiny hair, glowing skin, and a healthy weight.

Coconut oil itself does not contain cholesterol, but it does support healthy cholesterol formation in the liver. It raises levels of high-density lipoprotein (HDL), which is essential to healthy hormone production. It converts HDL into pregnenolone, the precursor to many hormones, including progesterone, known as the "beauty hormone." Progesterone improves circulation to the skin, giving us a natural face-lift by tightening up our saggy places. It also counteracts fatigue and protects the nervous system from stress. Reduced progesterone levels in the body contribute to the physical aging process and, over time, cause us to look and feel haggard and run-down.

Much like grasses, coconut palms have the ability to absorb nearly every mineral from the soil and environment where they grow, so they grow best with ocean water as a fertilizer and produce epic coconuts when properly nourished.

Typically, coconut oil contains numerous medium-chain triglycerides (MCTs) that coincide with coconut oil's powerful antiviral, antifungal, and antimicrobial properties. The MCTs include caproic acid (C6), which converts easily to ketones for energy; caprylic (C8), which is antimicrobial and easily converted to energy; capric acid (C10), another antimicrobial, antifungal compound in coconut oil that is easily converted to energy; and antiviral lauric acid (C12), which sits on the fence between MCTs and LCTs (long-chain triglycerides). These MCTs are typically marketed as quick energy brain foods to be consumed with coffee in the morning to improve performance and brain acuity. Coconut oil applied to the skin or taken internally naturally supports the immune system to keep us healthy while reducing inflammation—two important pieces of the beauty puzzle.

I highly recommend using coconut oil as your cooking oil of choice. When you heat unsaturated oils (canola oil, corn oil, margarine, safflower oil, soy oil, vegetable oil, etc.) to high temperatures, they create highly toxic trans-fatty acids, which go to work in your system like a slow drip of poison set to ultimately destroy how you look, leading to wrinkles and liver spots. If the buildup of rancid oils continues, it causes damage to your major organs, like the heart and liver, which reduces their ability to absorb nutrients and filter out toxins, affecting your appearance even further.

Topically, coconut oil is amazing for everything from smoothing scars to moisturizing dry elbows. Here are some of the best uses of coconut oil on the skin:

- Cuticle oil
- Hair tamer
- Lip balm
- Makeup remover
- Shaving cream

How to Buy Coconut Oil and/or MCT Oil

It's important to look for coconut oil and/or MCT oil that is organic, cold-pressed, and stored in a glass bottle or jar. All oils, including coconut oil and MCT oil, are light sensitive. Keep oils away from the damaging spectrums of light and they will stay viable for at least two years. Be sure to seek out MCT oils that are free of solvents and oxygen damage.

GOJI BERRIES

The goji is likely the most nutritionally rich berry on earth, which is a tall title for such a small fruit. Goji berries grow on a bush that is incredibly hardy. The plant has the ability to grow prolifically in the harsh climate of a desert, in temperate climates where it snows all winter, and in humid tropical climates. This adaptability infuses the goji with a certain strength that has earned it the designation of "adaptogen." In the world of medicinal plants, this means the goji can both strengthen and support the body's systems while at the same time helping counteract stress.

The rich red-orange color of the goji gives a visual hint of its wealth of antioxidant properties. It typically contains two to four times more antioxidants than blueberries! Antioxidants pull the damaging effects of free radicals out of your system and keep your liver clean and functioning, which translates into clear, glowing skin and smooth, shiny hair.

The goji berry is a complete protein source; contains nineteen amino acids and all nine essential amino acids; boasts at least twenty-one trace minerals (including zinc, iron, copper, calcium, germanium, selenium, and phosphorus) as well as vitamins B_1, B_2, B_6, and E, and high levels of hydrogen. As I mentioned, it's incredibly high in anti-oxidants, like tetraterpenoids, carotenoids, and zeaxanthin. Plus, it contains sesquiterpenoids, beta-sitosterol, linoleic acid, betaine, and polysaccharides, all of which feed cells the exact nutrients they need to keep skin plump and healthy.

One unique nutritional factor of the goji is its ability to help stimulate the body to produce more human growth hormone (HGH). As the body ages, it produces less HGH. Lower HGH causes us to feel less energetic, experience muscle loss, and start storing more body fat. Goji berries are the only food known to naturally help stimulate the production of HGH.

Goji Schizandra Berry Lemonade

Serves 2

- **32 ounces spring water, chilled**
- **1 cup fresh or frozen raspberries (though any kind of berries can be used)**
- **Juice of 2 medium lemons**
- **1 tablespoon goji berries**
- **2 teaspoons schizandra berry powder**
- **Raw organic honey and/or stevia**
- **Pinch of sea salt**

Blend all the ingredients together in a high-speed blender and enjoy!

Optional: Add 2 teaspoons chia seeds or some fresh aloe vera gel to supercharge this great herbal tonic!

HEMP SEEDS AND SEED OIL

Hemp is hands down one of the best sources of complete bioavailable plant protein available to us! Hemp protein's beauty prowess lies in its makeup: 66 percent is edestin and 33 percent is albumin. Edestin is used by the body to create almost all types of enzymes, hormones, and blood molecules while it also contributes to stress reduction, all of which affect beauty. Albumin maintains the strength of tissues, which contributes to taut, smooth skin.

Oil from the hemp seed touts one of the highest percentages of essential fatty acids of nearly any seed on earth in an almost perfect ratio to meet the body's nutritional needs. EFAs are antioxidants that protect skin from sun damage and support the health of the brain, eyes, and cardiovascular system. They help the body burn excess fat and remove toxins from the skin, intestinal tract, kidneys, and lungs. Hemp oil is an outstanding source of omega-3 (alpha-linolenic acid [ALA]); omega-6 (linoleic acid and gamma-linoleic acid [GLA], an anti-inflammatory powerhouse that helps with hormone balance); and omega-9 (oleic acid), which is a clean energy source for the body and a quality beauty support for the skin.

Hemp's sulfur-containing amino acids, methionine and cysteine, aid enzyme formation and assist the liver in filtering out toxins; they also improve the immune system, physical strength, complexion, and the luster of both skin and hair, all while keeping the skin free of eczema, dryness, scaling, cracking, and some forms of acne.

As far as vitamins and minerals, hemp contains three times more vitamin E than flaxseeds, which the skin and hair love, and is a good source of brain-sustaining, liver-supporting, cell membrane–building lecithin. Hemp provides a burst of vitamins A, B, and D, and is one of the few seeds that contain chlorophyll in the amazing tiny green leaves that live within each seedpod. Excelling at absorbing minerals from the soil, hemp seeds offer an abundance of major minerals, more than twenty trace minerals, and what I consider to be the four essential beauty minerals: silicon, sulfur, zinc, and iron.

Topically, you can gently apply hemp oil to moisturize dry skin while firming and tightening its appearance. Many people don't like using oil on their face because it leaves their skin feeling greasy. Hemp oil can moisturize without clogging pores, is naturally calming to the skin, can reduce the appearance of fine lines and wrinkles, and is widely tolerated by all different skin types. You can even use hemp oil on your hair, as it's naturally conditioning without being heavy.

HONEY

For years, honey was my superfood of choice. While I was getting my mechanical engineering and political science degrees at UC Santa Barbara, I would sit and sip honey while taking tests, because the glucose in honey is the perfect brain food. I'm sure you can imagine the looks I got! It definitely looked weird, but, man, did I nail those tests! My brain was supercharged on honey, since all the body's cells are powered by the mitochondria within them, and mitochondria are fueled by sugars like the ones in honey.

Honey nourishes cells not only for brain-based activities but also for throat healing and burn healing. Honey is so important and valuable to me as a superfood energy source and topical skin repair and beautifier that I began producing our own NoniLand Honey at our NoniLand farm in Hawaii. In the beginning, in situations where industrial buildings or private homes wanted to remove or destroy beehives, my team and I would volunteer to rescue the unwanted beehives and bring them back to our research facility. We brought the hives back to my farm and started a bee sanctuary on my property. I now have more than a million bees living with me. Not only do they subsist on the wide variety of superfood and superherb plants and trees I grow—such as noni, cacao, vanilla, mango, avocado, coconut, banana, jackfruit, durian, soursop, rollinia, citrus fruits, black sapote, akee, and tulsi (which they *love*)—I also sometimes feed them super-foods, such as spirulina.

When applied topically, honey acts as a humectant, drawing water out of the air and into itself, making it intensely hydrating. In its raw, unfiltered, and preferably wild state, honey is rich in minerals, antioxidants, probiotics, enzymes, and antibacterial properties, which act to protect and nourish damaged skin. For these reasons, honey is used today as an ingredient in many beauty products.

Honey has gained acceptance in the treatment of ulcers and the topical treatment of bed sores and other skin infections that come about from burns and wounds, and it is now used to deal with infections on skin grafts and skin graft donor sites. It has been shown to rapidly clear infections from deep surgical wounds that aren't responding to antibiotics and antiseptics, including wounds infected with the methicillin-resistant bacteria *Staphylococcus aureus*.

Internally, raw honey supports the production of melatonin, which is essential for a good night's sleep, and sleep affects telomeres, a critical component of beauty and healthy aging. Honey's amino acids support tissue rebuilding and repair to keep the foundation under the skin plump and strong. In its raw unprocessed form, honey is one of nature's richest sources of live healing enzymes, containing about two hundred active substances on average. These enzymes make honey a nourishing replacement for white sugar and high-fructose corn syrup; they support digestion, the assimilation of food and nutrients, and weight loss efforts (unlike fake sweeteners, which tear your body down and create fat).

The composition of honey varies a bit, depending on the plants the bees visit. However, almost all natural honey is composed primarily of fructose and glucose, and contains fructooligosaccharides, lots of amino acids, vitamins, minerals, enzymes, phenolics, peptides, flavonoids, phenolic acids, tocopherols, and superoxide dismutase, which work together to heal the body both inside and out. All of these factors together make honey such an all-around medicinal superstar superfood.

How can you leverage the mighty antioxidant effects of honey on your skin? Here are my top three topical ways to reduce acne, hydrate your skin, boost your complexion, and get that coveted glow so many chemical beauty products pretend to offer.

Moisturizing mask: Dampen your face with warm water, then apply about half a teaspoon of raw honey in a thin layer, massaging your skin in a circular motion. Leave the honey on your face for at least thirty minutes. Rinse it off with warm water, and be prepared for soft, radiant skin.

Zit zapper: Don't reach for an over-the-counter acne remedy when you pop out with an annoying blemish. Instead, dab a little raw honey on the offender before you go to sleep. (Make sure your fingertip is clean when you apply it!) In the morning, you'll notice your skin will be less annoyed with you and well on its way to recovery. If you have a major zit forming, mix the honey with 1 drop lavender essential oil before you apply it. If the blemish is threatening to take over your face, mix the honey with 1 drop each lavender and tea tree essential oils, and knock that monster down.

Pore empowerer: Let the enzymes in raw honey do the dirty work to get the gunk out of your pores. Mix 1 tablespoon raw honey with 2 tablespoons coconut oil until they are well combined. Wash your face with warm water, dry it well, then apply the honey-and-coconut-oil mixture, massaging it into your skin using circular motions while avoiding the eye area. Let the mixture sit for a few minutes before rinsing it off with lukewarm water.

What Kind of Honey Should You Buy?

Buy only raw, unprocessed, organic honey. The golden, syrup-like honey you see around in the cute little bears has been heavily processed, chemically refined, or heat-treated, which destroys the beneficial enzymes, vitamins, and minerals.

MACA

Maca is a member of the cruciferous family, alongside its crunchy cousins broccoli, cabbage, cauliflower, kale, radishes, and turnips. Maca is cultivated for its root, which comes in different colors— off-white, yellow, red, purple, or black—and is traditionally dried, powdered, and/or cooked. The dried root tastes slightly malty with butterscotch overtones, so it works easily into smoothies, teas, nut milks, and coffee. It also pairs well with my buddy cacao. (Superfood chocolate "malted milkshakes" are the best ever!)

For approximately 2,600 years, maca has thrived high in the Peruvian Andes of South America. Today, maca is still the highest altitude crop on earth and is cultivated by descendants of the Incas at altitudes between 9,000 and 14,000 feet (about 2,700 and 4,300 meters) above sea level. Its growing region is intense, barren, and inhospitable. In the face of such extremes, this plant has developed incredibly powerful adaptogenic properties.

Maca has the ability to balance your glandular-hormonal system, nervous system, cardiovascular system, and musculature. It also works to make your body adaptable to stressful situations. It acts on the adrenals to provide you with energy while at the same time keeping you calm and levelheaded. Maca shows promise for stress management, and studies show that maca supplementation can reduce anxiety and even help fight depression. As you know, stress is

EATING SEASONALLY

Eating seasonally is an ancient Ayurvedic method for optimizing nutrition, radiant health, and beauty. Eating foods that are in harmony with the season syncs the body with its immediate environment and maximizes what nature provides. Eating out of season is common practice, but we have not stopped to consider if this is actually the best thing for our health and physical vitality.

Fortunately, nature in its infinite wisdom makes it extremely easy to eat in season, because all foods are perfectly timed and ideal for our health in the season they grow in. No matter what country or climate you live in, nature provides you with the ideal food to eat at any given time.

Remember your body's rhythm is connected to the rhythm of each day and night and also the seasonal flow of the environment in which you live. By adopting a natural diet in alignment with your environment you will harness the power of Mother Nature and deliver efficient nutrition to every cell of your body. In addition, eating in season is less expensive and has a lower carbon footprint, and foods in season are fresher and tastier because they are picked on time and not before they are ripe.

a beauty killer, so maca is a potent ally in your war against stress.

The libido- and fertility-enhancing properties of maca are due to its action on the hypothalamus, the sex-hormone center of the brain. The hypothalamus stimulates the pituitary gland to secrete luteinizing hormone and follicle-stimulating hormone, which in turn stimulate the adrenal glands and gonads to secrete testosterone, progesterone, and dehydroepiandrosterone (DHEA).

Why is this important? As you become overburdened with toxins, demineralized, and suffer from poor nutrition, you produce less of these hormones. This decrease in hormones causes the physical signs of aging. Therefore increasing hormone production naturally with maca can keep your body looking younger longer. Fortunately, since maca is an adaptogen, it will keep your hormones in check, leveling them out only when needed.

Maca is composed of around 76 percent carbohydrates, 8 percent fiber, 5 percent fat, and slightly more than 10 percent protein. Although it is not a complete protein, it contains twenty amino acids, including seven of the essential ones. It is such an outstanding source of hormone precursors that it provides many of the same effects high-protein foods typically provide to boost the shine of your hair and to strengthen your nails.

Maca also offers macro- and micronutrients, including thirty-one different minerals to optimize cellular function. Two of my favorite beauty minerals are iron and iodine, which are important to note because they support your thyroid. When your thyroid isn't functioning properly, it leads to hair thinning and sallow skin. Maca can play an important role in strengthening your mane and maintaining youthful skin tone.

Also note that maca is best taken in cycles. Include it three weeks during the month, then take the next week off for maximum effectiveness. (The following tonic includes chaga, which you can learn more about on page 164.)

Macagenic Tonic

A delicious adaptogenic superfood beverage with maca.

    2 cups warm chaga tea

    1 tablespoon cacao powder

    1 tablespoon protein powder

    1 tablespoon coconut oil

1 tablespoon raw organic honey

2 teaspoons maca powder

½ teaspoon ground cinnamon

¼ teaspoon vanilla powder

½ squirt English Toffee stevia

Pinch of sea salt

Make sure your chaga tea has been strained of any leftover chaga pieces, then blend the filtered tea with all the other ingredients in a high-speed blender and enjoy!

OLIVE OIL

Olive oil is lubricating, cleansing, beautifying, and rejuvenating. It can be eaten as well as applied topically, and its elite nutritional content makes it a superfood of the highest order.

Olive oil is what I like to call a "good" fat. The largest component of olive oil—between 55 and 85 percent—is the beautifying monounsaturated fat oleic acid. At the cellular level, oleic acid is used by the plasma membranes to remain fluid and soft. These cell membranes are made up of large amounts of fat and cholesterol, and when your diet contains high amounts of oleic acid, your cell membranes are more resistant to oxidation, slowing down the aging process.

Oleic acid is a superstar at reducing bad cholesterol too, and regular consumption of olive oil has been shown to protect against coronary heart disease by decreasing arterial clogging. When blood can flow freely, it nourishes cells and the skin radiates a clear level of beauty.

Olives and their oil contain an abundance of vitamin E, which is known to erase fine lines on the face and repair connective tissue.

Vitamin E also plays a role in the health of the circulatory system and is incredibly soothing to the digestive tract. The beauty-enhancing substance squalene (one of the most common oils produced by human skin cells) is found within olive oil as well. This is noteworthy because as it smooths the appearance of your skin it also offers a nice boost to your immune system.

It's important to eat olive oil raw or apply it directly to your skin, because cooked oil and cooked fats are the most detrimental of all foods to physical beauty. They are inflammatory to tissues, clog the cardiovascular system, and accelerate the cellular aging process. They destroy the complexion and lead to face and body acne. Raw oil, however, does exactly the opposite. Raw fats and oils are some of the best foods to include in your diet, because they beautify the skin, lubricate the joints and intestines, strengthen cell membranes, fight inflammation, and restore fat-soluble nutrients to the tissues.

How to Pick a Good-Quality Olive Oil

Look for an organic stone-crushed or cold-pressed extra-virgin oil sold in a dark glass bottle. Oils are light sensitive and should never be kept in a clear glass or plastic-leaching bottle.

PUMPKIN SEEDS AND SEED OIL

Besides having an awesomely delicious rich nutty flavor, pumpkin seed oil is an anti-aging superpower packed with nutrition. It's a wonderful source of B and E vitamins, many minerals like zinc and magnesium, phytonutrients (cucurbitin, phytosterol), and essential fatty acids. It contains hormone-building elements that support a healthy libido and sexual function as well as myosin, the chief protein constituent of nearly all the muscles in the body. The seeds also have vitamin B_{17}, otherwise known as laetrile or amygdalin, which has reputed antitumor effects.

Raw pumpkin seeds are one of the best sources of the amino acid tryptophan too. This amino acid is often lacking in people's diets because it is intolerant to high heat and is destroyed by cooking. Tryptophan works with tyrosine and zinc to elevate one's mood and increase levels of serotonin in the brain, alleviating depression and brain chemistry imbalances caused by using drugs, such as MDMA (Ecstasy), that deplete the adrenal system. Tryptophan's relaxing qualities also help alleviate stress and insomnia.

Pumpkin seed oil assists with detoxification since raw pumpkin seeds contain high concentrations of methionine, popularly recognized for its power to draw heavy metals out of the body. Sulfur, the foundational mineral of all beauty, is also found in the methionine in pumpkin seeds. Sulfur produces a rosy complexion and has been recognized for centuries for its contribution to natural beauty.

Pumpkin seeds are an excellent source of unsaturated fatty acids as well, including oleic fatty acid, along with omega-6 and trace amounts of omega-3. Oleic acid has strong beautifying properties, lowers blood pressure, and adds extra protection from sunburn.

The anti-inflammatory, antioxidant nutrients in pumpkin seeds (and all members of the cucumber family) help with dark circles under the eyes and support hydrated, clear, radiant skin.

Pumpkin seed oil supports new hair growth and is especially helpful for men dealing with male-pattern baldness. In a recent study, men who took 400 milligrams of pumpkin seed oil every day for twenty-four weeks actually had 40 percent more hair growth than men in the placebo group, with no adverse effects whatsoever!

This amazing seed oil can be used in raw-food recipes and on salads, and, like most superfoods, it can be used topically to maximize its medicinal and beautifying properties. Apply it directly on the scalp, to help condition hair, or the skin, as a healing salve for burns and wounds and to improve overall skin tone and appearance.

This dark green, flavor-rich, detoxifying, beautifying, medicinally beneficial super oil is best when it is cold-pressed. Store it in a dark container in a cool spot out of direct sunlight to prevent oxidation.

SPIRULINA

It's not easy being green . . . unless you're spirulina, and then it's pretty awesome since you're the most powerful single-celled super-food swimming in the earth's volcanic waters.

Since the dawn of time, this microscopic, freshwater algae has helped sustain the earth's food chain by providing fundamental nutrition for all sources of life. Spirulina has been around since life first appeared on earth, and it is the foundation of the food chain as we know it. For several thousand years, ancient civilizations depended on spirulina as their primary protein source.

At least thirty-five varieties of spirulina exist today. They are incredibly hardy—some are able to stay alive in a dormant state when water evaporates or when they are exposed to high temperatures during travel and food processing. Even under such extreme circumstances, they retain their nutrients. Spirulina is so rich in nutrition that you could potentially live on it alone for quite a long time if you needed to.

Although tiny, spirulina sports a whopping 65 to 71 percent protein, the highest concentration by weight of any food available. It's a complete protein and contains all nine essential amino acids. Spirulina is easier for the body to digest and assimilate than beef and contains at least twice the protein.

As such, it's a builder of lean muscle and an aid to your skin's collagen and elastin levels. It's the only green food that contains the superstar gamma-linoleic acid, which reduces inflammation and supports healthy hormone production.

A fantastic source of carotenoids and phytonutrient antioxidants, spirulina wages a heavy war against the damaging effects of free radicals on your appearance. It can help prevent the wrinkling, sagging, and discoloration that occurs when too many free radicals build up in your system from sun exposure, air pollution, and poor diet. It also contains the antioxidant zeaxanthin, which is potent in maintaining the health of your eyes, and superoxide dismutase, one of the most health-enhancing metabolic enzymes you can consume since it helps all cells function at their best.

One more important antioxidant spirulina touts is the gorgeous bluish-green protein pigment phycocyanin, which contributes to spirulina's famous color. Phycocyanin stimulates the production of stem cells. These cells replace aging skin cells, and maintaining and protecting production of them is key to keeping the skin elastic, moisturized, and wrinkle-free as long as possible. When skin cells turn over faster, we maintain a healthy glow, because old skin cells make us look dry and dull.

Walking hand in hand with antioxidants, the green pigment chlorophyll is in high concentrations in spirulina, making it one of nature's most cleansing foods. Detoxing the junk out of our cells, like heavy metals and other environmental toxins, keeps the skin clear, the eyes bright, and the body's weight in check. Chlorophyll is also an excellent blood builder, ensuring that toxins are carried out of the system so they don't just get recycled and stuck in the organs.

One more robust beauty enhancer spirulina offers is bioavailable sulfur. It actually contains several kinds of sulfur, which improves the immune system, liver function, physical strength, tissue repair, complexion, and hair luster. Sulfur also helps regulate the sodium–

potassium electrolyte balance in and out of the body's cells, so all cells can work together to the best of their ability.

Try blending spirulina into fresh juices, salad dressings, or your favorite smoothie. It tastes amazing sprinkled on organic, non-GMO popcorn with coconut oil and Icelandic sea salt. It is also outstanding when applied topically in a face mask.

Very Green Drink

There are few things better for you on God's green earth than green foods! Greens contain chlorophyll, the component in plants that absorbs energy from the sun to facilitate photosynthesis. Chlorophyll is to plants what blood is to humans, so ingesting chlorophyll is like getting a transfusion of sorts! When you eat densely green superfoods, you get all the benefits of chlorophyll at the cellular level plus other amazing nutrients that help to detoxify, energize, and mineralize the body. So don't forget to drink your greens!

8 ounces coconut milk, chilled

3 tablespoons tocotrienols (rice bran solubles)

1 tablespoon coconut oil, melted

1 tablespoon maca powder

1 tablespoon almond butter

1 to 2 teaspoons spirulina

1 teaspoon chlorella powder

20 fresh mint leaves

Raw organic honey

Ice (optional)

Blend all the ingredients together in a high-speed blender and enjoy cold!

SUPERHERBS

In my decades of research, I have discovered, grown, and worked with a class of unsurpassed herbs so efficacious that I classify them as superherbs. Superherbs possess an astonishing array of highly nutritional components, including antioxidants, saponins, polysaccharides, enzymes, medicinal color pigments, vitamins, trace minerals, and more. They are backed by thousands of years of proven use in the systems of Chinese and Ayurvedic herbalism. I firmly believe that superherbs have the ability to vastly improve our health and enhance our beauty, promoting lustrous hair, radiant skin, strong nails, and a beautiful smile!

Members of ancient civilizations, such as the Chinese Taoists, European alchemists, Mayan priest-kings, and Indian yogis, did not need microscopes and cellular viewpoints as proof; their superherb use was (and is) based on physical experiences and time-tested strategies and intuition—which we should all appreciate.

CHINESE TONIC HERBALISM: FIVE THOUSAND YEARS OF HEALTH AND HEALING

The most powerful system for enhancing beauty and health is found in Traditional Chinese Medicine (TCM). For centuries Chinese women have had an uncanny ability to halt aging in its tracks. These beauty secrets are now available to us, and the discovery of Chinese tonic herbalism was a pivotal moment in my life. I consistently rely upon tonic herbs as much as any superfood. They are a cornerstone of my diet. By exploring the basic principles of jing, chi, and shen, I learned to extract the underlying causes and conditions of beauty and further

stack the deck in my favor. And I am going to share some of these
secrets with you.

Jing, chi, and shen are three vital energies, or forces in nature and
within the human body itself, that determine our physical health,
energy, and mental state. These three health-giving energies ultimately determine how we look and feel. The traditional analogy
comparing these energies to a candle is that jing is the wax, chi is the
flame, and shen is the light emitted by the flame.

Jing is the physical essence that determines how long we live. It is our
deepest energy store, or our lifelong core battery. It is located in the
kidneys and is often referred to as "kidney essence." We are born with
a finite amount of jing, received primarily from our mother. If jing
becomes severely depleted, then sickness and death are imminent.
The key to beauty and health is to maintain our jing as long as possible and only dip into our jing "bank account" in extreme emergen-
cies. The body's ability to repair and rejuvenate is dependent on jing
reserves. As jing wanes, the body cannot push back on the ravaging
effects of aging. Gray hair, wrinkled, sagging, dry skin, and distortion
of our figure begin to occur, and the best we are able to do is cover and
conceal. The first step in TCM is to stop "leaking" jing, because this is
akin to letting your life force slip away. The jing-nourishing herbs are
the most coveted in Chinese medicine. When we consume them, we
are literally adding days to our life.

My favorite jing-nourishing superherbs and special foods (in both
the Chinese system and other systems) include the following:

- Black foods: black beans, blackberry, black (cumin) seed oil, black
  currant, black honey, black maca, black mulberry, black olives
  (not treated with ferrous gluconate), black radish, black rice, black
  seaweeds (e.g., bladderwrack, nori), black sesame seed, black
  walnut hull

- Black supplements: activated charcoal, charcoal, shilajit
- Chaga mushroom
- Cistanche
- Cordyceps
- Eucommia bark
- He shou wu
- Mature aged ginseng
- Rehmannia root
- Schizandra

Chi is our ability to mobilize energy. It is the energy we take in from breathing and eating and the energy currency we work with on a day-to-day basis. From a beauty perspective, chi is incredibly important, because chi is involved in moving toxins out of the body and delivering nutrients from the blood to the skin. Plus, chi determines the vibrancy of our cells. Clear eyes, glowing skin, and overall radiance are signs that chi is flowing nicely.

My favorite chi-nourishing superherbs and special foods (in both the Chinese system and other systems) include the following:

- Amla
- Ashwagandha
- Astragalus
- Citrus peel (breaks up stagnation)
- Dong quai
- Gac fruit (Vietnamese lycopene-rich superfruit)
- Ginseng
- Goji berries
- Gynostemma
- Jujube
- Longan fruit
- Neem

- Red foods: beets, blood orange, chard, cherries, cranberry, dragon fruit (pitaya), hawthorn berries, plums, pomegranate, radishes, red apples, red berries (raspberry, strawberry, etc.), red chilies, red maca, red peppers, red rice, rhubarb, tomatoes, watermelon
- Red supplements: red clay (great topically), red salt (alaea)
- Reishi mushroom
- Schizandra

Shen is our aura—our spiritual presence. Shen may be thought of as arising naturally from strong jing and flowing chi. It is the mental and spiritual state that accompanies great health and a clean body. Shen incorporates the intangible qualities that make someone attractive. The grace, patience, and goodwill that radiates from a person with strong shen is hard to miss.

My favorite shen-nourishing superherbs and special foods (in both the Chinese system and other systems) include the following:
- Albizia flower
- Asparagus root (shatavari)
- Codonopsis root
- Pearl
- Reishi mushroom
- Royal jelly (queen bee food)
- Shen foods: homegrown foods, wild foods, wild mushrooms
- Shen supplements: betaine (not betaine hydrochloride), charcoal, MSM (methyl-sulfonyl methane)
- White peony root

The vibration achieved through the cultivation of the three treasures of jing, chi, and shen is the essence of beauty—not only physical beauty but also a beautiful way of being. The most important aspect of cultivating jing, chi, and shen is balance. If we oscillate between stagnation and overexercise, eating clean and bingeing on processed foods and cooked unsaturated oils, shallow breathing and two-hour yoga classes, we will find it impossible to maintain beauty during middle and old age. However, when we maintain a consistent balance day in and day out, we don't engage in frantic overcompensation, which seems to be the hallmark of a Western approach to health and beauty.

Incorporating superherbs into your diet is easy. These substances have innate intelligence and will influence you in profound ways, enabling you to activate your body's ability to experience the radiant health that is your birthright.

The Top Ten Superherbs for Beauty

- Amla
- Ashwagandha
- Asparagus root
- He shou wu
- Longan berry
- Neem
- Pearl
- Schizandra
- Tulsi
- White peony root

AMLA

Known as "the rejuvenator," "the sustainer," or the Indian gooseberry, amla is a plant that has been widely used within the five-thousand-year-old Indian Ayurvedic system, including in hair oils, hair thickeners, and shampoos. The Indian gooseberry is believed to be a tree of enlightenment in Hindu mythology, given to enhance health and lengthen life.

Whether you eat it, drink it, or apply it topically, amla is a potent skin enhancer. It's rich in superoxide dismutase and antioxidants, which reduce the signs of premature aging and pigmentation, like fine lines, wrinkles, and age spots. The antioxidants, in combination with mega doses of vitamin C (ten times more than oranges!), lend a brightness to the skin while toning and tightening it. These properties also help protect the skin from harmful UV rays and boost collagen production, keeping skin looking youthful. Amla paste can be applied topically as an effective treatment against acne and scar spots, and amla juice can be used as an exfoliant to remove dead skin cells.

Not only does amla benefit your skin, it's equally fantastic for your hair. As a rich source of essential fatty acids, it nourishes your hair, starting at the roots. The antioxidants in amla oil stop premature graying and thicken up your hair nicely. Drinking amla juice improves the health of your scalp, knocking out dandruff, and it's known to make hair shinier. Amla paste can be applied directly to heal split ends or rubbed into the scalp to reduce hair loss.

As if that's not enough, by increasing your protein levels, amla helps your body burn fat faster. If your breath is a little less than sweet, or if you have bleeding gums, gargling with amla can bring your mouth pH into balance. You can also use amla pulp as a toothpaste due to its antibacterial and astringent qualities.

ASHWAGANDHA

In Sanskrit, "ashwagandha" means "smell of a horse," but don't let this translation turn you away from incorporating this stress-reducing superherb into your lifestyle. Good news: it doesn't actually smell that bad. Its name references the power of the plant to impart horse-like strength and energy to the one who eats it.

All parts of the plant can be used medicinally for different purposes, with the root being the main powerhouse. If you can add only one superherb to your arsenal at a time, ashwagandha is the perfect one to start with, because it's a total-body herb that positively affects almost every beauty factor I talk about in this book.

Ashwagandha contains a high amount of antioxidants. It helps your hair maintain strength and shine, making it less prone to damage, and the anti-inflammatory properties of the herb work against scalp conditions, like dandruff, scalp psoriasis, greasy hair, and eczema. The tyrosine in ashwagandha boosts the production of melanin in hair, which combats premature graying; it is even used in some shampoos because it improves circulation to the scalp, accelerating hair growth. This fights the good fight against androgenetic alopecia, otherwise known as balding.

Ayurvedic practitioners have long recommended using ashwagandha against acne and other inflammatory skin conditions. It fights the signs of skin aging, like wrinkles, dark spots, and fine lines. Topical oils or pastes made from the leaves and roots can treat painful skin swelling and help irritated skin heal faster.

With its antibacterial and antifungal properties, ashwagandha is an incredible support to the immune system and is known to increase the production of white blood cells, keeping the body strong against invaders. It also helps improve digestion, flushing toxins out of the body, keeping the liver clean.

ASPARAGUS ROOT

This root doesn't come from the asparagus you can grab off your local grocery store shelf or harvest out of your garden, the official name of which is *Asparagus officinalis*. Instead, it comes from a wild asparagus plant (*Asparagus cochinchinensis*). Wild asparagus root is a special herb that has been revered in China for over two thousand years for its medicinal qualities.

Asparagus root is a strong cleanser for the lungs, liver, and blood.

It's packed with vitamins, minerals, and phytonutrients that promote smooth, supple, soft skin and can effectively treat blemishes. It provides rich stores of vitamins C and E, which can boost the production of collagen, a vital component of connective tissues, and it can nourish and protect skin from dryness. It also works to strengthen the roots of hair and to moisturize the scalp.

Taoists believe the consumption of this herb can give you the ability to fly! Of course, it doesn't really help you fly but rather symbolizes the ability to rise above things that are mundane, helping you to achieve harmony in all that you do. Asparagus root is said to increase feelings of compassion, joy, and happiness while reducing stress and anxiety. Many say taking asparagus root opens the heart center, and aren't we all more beautiful when we learn to live through the heart?

HE SHOU WU

He shou wu (aka ho shou wu) is the root of the plant *Polygonum multiflorum* and has been used for centuries in Traditional Chinese Medicine as a blood-building, sexuality-enhancing, rejuvenating beauty superherb.

One of the most famous attributes of he shou wu is its proclaimed ability to turn gray hair back to its original dark color. In fact, "he shou wu" literally means "old black-haired man." As the body ages, it conserves resources and energy and redirects them to its vital functions. The nonessential functions, like maintaining hair and nail quality, decline faster than other functions simply because they are not needed to keep the body alive. He shou wu strengthens the kidneys and liver to such an extent that the body can redirect energy into maintaining the color and health of hair, skin, and nails.

Strengthening the kidneys and liver also promotes better detoxification, allowing for a more effective process of flushing toxins, which contribute to aging.

Known for its influence on the circulatory system, he shou wu can induce an expansion of the blood vessels (vasodilation), allowing nutrient delivery to happen more efficiently and on a larger scale throughout the body. This, along with he shou wu's high levels of zinc, supports maximum cellular proficiency and, in particular, muscle growth and recovery.

In Chinese herbalism, he shou wu is also revered for its stamina-boosting, aphrodisiac properties and has been used to treat infertility and a low libido. This is most likely due to its ability to stimulate hormones, such as estrogen, human growth hormone, cortisol, and testosterone. Its effect on hormones also calms hyperactive adrenals and balances cortisol, which can contribute to reducing belly fat.

Consuming he shou wu is easy. I use it as a base for many of my teas, as it has a pleasant, earthy flavor. When you combine it in a tea with other superherbs, you enter into the upper levels of beauty protocols. These were the very herbs consumed for thousands of years by sages, imperial courts, and men and women whose lives were dedicated to the mastery of youth and longevity.

LONGAN BERRY

Native to southern China, longan berry is called *long yan rou* in Chinese, which translates to "dragon eye meat." Longan berry obviously isn't meat or a dragon's eye; rather, the name describes the interior of the fruit, where a soft orb of translucent flesh surrounds a dark black pit. Longan berry has been used in tonic herbalism for about two thousand years as both a dried fruit and a raw food to support the cardiovascular system, supply energy, cultivate beautiful skin, reduce anxiety and stress, and promote healthy sleep cycles. I have grown longan berry for years and I am impressed by its toughness! Through drought or downpour from Los Angeles to Hawaii to China, longan berry thrives.

Longan berry is a cardiovascular supporter of the highest order. Its blood-building properties come from its high organic iron content. It offers more than twenty times the iron of grapes and fifteen times the iron of spinach! What's even better is the body can regulate how much of this iron it needs since it's an organic form of iron. This means that men, who generally need less iron than women, won't get constipated from absorbing too much iron, while women will have ample iron available to support their menstrual cycle and add luster to their skin and hair. All of this available iron works to improve blood circulation, allowing toxins to move out of the system with ease and minerals and vitamins to get where they need to go.

If you're looking for a food to supply you with at least 80 percent of your daily vitamin C requirement, then longan berry is the clear choice. The vitamin C helps your body soak up the iron it needs more easily and, of course, boosts your immune system to fight off bacteria and viruses. Vitamin C, in combination with vitamin B, which longan also offers, protects your cells from free-radical damage and improves the appearance of skin tone, especially around the eyes. This fantastic food also keeps your teeth and gums healthy and sparkling.

Longan berry contains phosphorus, magnesium, potassium, and vitamin A as well as complex carbohydrates, giving you energy and reducing food cravings. So not only does it keep you glowing on the outside; it helps to keep your weight in check too.

Altogether, longan berry's components have a general calming effect on the body, which can help relieve stress and anxiety. It is also known to help induce sleep and allow us to sleep deeper—and, as we know, stress reduction and better sleep are significant keys to beauty.

NEEM

Neem has been a cornerstone of India's long-standing beauty tradition for centuries. Citizens would bathe with neem leaves to keep their skin healthy, crush leaves into face masks for emollient and anti-aging properties, apply neem leaf extract to acne and breakouts, and chew on neem twigs to keep their teeth disease free. Neem oil, extracted from the tree's seeds, has been revered for its medicinal properties in Ayurveda for more than four thousand years.

Skin does a happy dance when neem is applied to it because of the abundance of fatty acids, like oleic acid and linoleic acid, as well as vitamin E. Linoleic acid keeps the skin clear by preventing acne breakouts. Oleic acid is used by cell plasma membranes to resist oxidation, maintaining soft skin. Vitamin E acts as a free-radical scavenger, hindering damaging oxidative processes in the skin. Together, the fatty acids and vitamin E have the ability to rejuvenate skin cells. They penetrate deep to restore elasticity, heal scars, reduce wrinkles and fine lines, minimize pores, and reverse skin damage.

Neem is packed with antibacterial, antifungal, antiparasitic, anti-inflammatory, and antiseptic properties that make it excellent for solving the common beauty problems of acne, eczema, psoriasis, and more. It is unique in that it kills unwanted bacteria while leaving healthy and beneficial bacteria unharmed, making it a secret weapon in dental care. It can be an ally against dandruff and head lice too without the need to rely on chemical-laden shampoos. It also contains vitamin C, which helps remove blackheads from the skin, promotes normal pigmentation, prevents dullness, and can bring back the skin's youthful and radiant glow.

Neem leaf is very potent, and neem seed oil is both potent and pungent. To ingest neem leaf powder, start out with an encapsulated product. To put it on the skin, use bulk neem leaf powder in a skin formula or use neem seed oil in a carrier oil, like coconut oil, so you can dilute it.

I was so blown away when I learned about neem that I decided to start growing it. Now I have neem trees all over my property and firmly believe, after working with it for this long, that it is one of the great beauty herbs of the world. Here are a few ways I've discovered to use neem.

Dandruff controller: Warm 1 teaspoon neem oil with 1 teaspoon coconut oil and massage the mixture into your scalp. Wash it off after half an hour. Please note, it is completely safe—and more potent—to rub neem oil into your scalp without coconut oil if your skin can tolerate it.

Acne buster: Warm 1 teaspoon coconut oil or olive oil with 10 drops neem oil. Apply the mixture to the face and wash it off after an hour. If your skin tolerates neem well, you can leave it on overnight.

Face mask: Mix 2 teaspoons neem powder with 1 teaspoon coconut oil to improve dry skin, remove blackheads, shrink large pores, and get rid of whiteheads. Apply the mixture to your skin using circular motions and let it sit on your skin for 15 minutes before rinsing it off with cool water. You may substitute honey or yogurt for the coconut oil if you prefer, and for added effect, you can include ground turmeric or (my personal favorite) tulsi, also known as holy basil.

Bath booster: Add 2 to 5 full droppers (not drops) of neem alcohol tincture to your bathwater. Repeat this daily for one week and you should see fantastic results, particularly in the reduction of body acne or skin infection.

Dental assistant: Start using neem-based toothpaste. For a stronger dental health aid, rub neem oil directly onto the gums, let sit for a few minutes, then wash out with water. Neem seed oil is pungent, but you may find over time that you enjoy the smell and taste.

PEARL

In centuries past, an oyster would die in the process of extracting its pearl, but now, technology allows the oyster to live out its twelve-year life span while producing three to four pearls. Pearl is one of our top ten superherbs for good reason. It was used by the emperors and empresses of ancient China for well over two thousand years, both topically in face masks as well as internally for enriching the skin and preserving a youthful appearance.

Pearl has a direct affect upon the skin and liver due to its rich stores of bioavailable calcium. This is not the calcium found in most dietary supplements, which unfortunately is inflammatory and causes us to age faster. Most supplements contain positively charged calcium, which deposits in the body like sediment rather than being absorbed to help the bones. Negatively charged calcium—like what is found in plants and in pearl—is beneficial to consume because the body can absorb and use it.

Pearl also contains trace minerals essential for radiant skin, such as magnesium, zinc, iron, copper, selenium, and silicon.

The technology exists today to make pearl powder that is finely ground and easily absorbable, both internally and externally. If you have acne scars or damaged skin, a topical application of pearl can work wonders. If you experience regular red blotches on your skin, then pearl will help. Red, blotchy skin is often caused by excess heat in the liver, and pearl cools and calms the liver.

Pearl contains the blue pigment conchiolin. Conchiolin is pearl's secret weapon. Conchiolin acts like keratin (fibrous structural proteins and collagen found in skin, bone, nails, cartilage, tendons, hair, and so on), which may be what makes it beneficial to our skin and bones. It is now theorized that conchiolin performs like (or changes into) human collagen that then begins the formation of hydroxylapatite crystals, a naturally occurring form of calcium. The mineral compound, hydroxylapatite, can be found in teeth, enamel, dentin, and bones. Pearl should be consumed by women to protect their bones into menopause and beyond.

Pearl stimulates the production of superoxide dismutase (SOD), one of the most important antioxidants made by your body. Have you ever wondered why some people eat whatever they want, smoke, drink, and still look amazing? This is SOD in action. SOD is an enzyme that neutralizes oxidation and acts as your body's internal defense against aging, skin spots, and premature wrinkles.

Pearl has an added benefit with its dual directional activity, meaning it can supply you with energy during the day and calm you down at night. In fact, women in China enjoy pearl in the morning to perk themselves up, and give it to their children at night to ready them for sleep. Try the "Restore Your Radiance Pearl Replenisher" recipe on page 247 for a great drink to prepare you for the restorative beauty processes that happen during sleep!

SCHIZANDRA

Schizandra is used in many beauty products for its rejuvenating and restorative properties. The schizandra berry is most often associated with the Taoist goddess Magu, a Chinese deity who represents eternal beauty. I could honestly write a whole book about schizandra, it is so extraordinary, and it is one of my absolute favorite superherbs!

The Chinese name for schizandra is *wu wei zi,* which means "the five-flavored fruit." This is because schizandra contains all five tastes: sweet, sour, salty, bitter, and pungent (umami). From a beauty perspective, schizandra has the ability to cleanse the liver and purify the blood. In fact, it is both a phase I and phase II liver detoxifier, which means it helps break down toxins as well as helps the body eliminate them. (See the "Liver Detoxification" section on page 112 for more information.) Schizandra also acts as a natural skin moisturizer, *from the inside.* One of the reasons the skin dries out and wrinkles as we age is that the body has a greater difficulty holding on to moisture on a cellular level. By using schizandra, we can maintain juicier tissues and well-hydrated skin.

Schizandra falls into the tonic herb class due to its potency and can therefore be taken daily in powder or extract form. It is said to also protect the skin from wind damage and harsh external elements. (Try the Deluxe Schizandra and Berry Beauty Lemonade in the "Tonics" section of recipes, page 250.)

TULSI

Tulsi, also known as holy basil, is worshipped in India as the "mother medicine of nature" and is called the "queen of herbs." It has been used for over five thousand years as an important component of the Ayurvedic tradition for everything from quieting a cough to combating infection. This sacred herb is found in most Indian households and can be taken in many different forms, including eating the fresh leaves, drinking herbal teas, ingesting it as a dried powder, or applying it topically.

Tulsi has been one of my absolute favorite superherbs to grow. I originally planted one type of holy basil right near my house, because Ayurvedic tradition recommends it at the front of the house to act as a protector plant. Over the years, this holy basil has moved itself around the property! I'm not even kidding—I've never seen a plant do this. It would seed itself, then decide it didn't like that spot and seed somewhere else. Then it would decide it didn't like that spot either and would seed somewhere else. Eventually it ended up down near the end of the driveway, where it has happily remained in the same spot, growing bigger and bigger, for the past five years. Tulsi is truly one of those mysteries I can't explain, but in Ayurvedic traditions, holy basil is said to have a consciousness, and after my experience, I can't say I disagree with that! What I do know is I get holy basil into my body every single day, and let me tell you why.

Holy basil is an adaptogen that contains hundreds of beneficial components, including strong antioxidants and terpenes with anti-bacterial, antiviral, anti-inflammatory, and antiseptic properties. Tulsi is a premium disinfectant that rids the body of toxins, infections, and viral agents. It strengthens the kidneys to help filter out contaminants, boosts the circulatory system to reduce blood pressure and bad cholesterol levels, strengthens the digestive system to reduce bloating and constipation, and calms the nervous system to reduce stress.

These same antioxidants protect the skin by maintaining skin tone, cleaning out pores, tightening, and repairing. The flavonoids orientin and vicenin in tulsi protect chromosomes from oxidation. This blocks damage from occurring to cells, which causes the visual appearance of aging. When applied topically, tulsi can eliminate fine lines around the eyes, and when taken internally, it can help to keep eyesight from degenerating. Its purifying qualities make it a world-class acne buster and eczema healer too.

Let's not forget about your smile! Tulsi is a power player in the mouth. It acts as an oral disinfectant for the teeth and gums as well as a natural breath freshener and teeth whitener.

WHITE PEONY ROOT

There is an old Chinese saying: "A woman who consumes peony root will become as beautiful as the peony flower itself." This beauty-supporting plant has been cultivated in China since 900 BCE and was even named as the national flower of China. It is the three- and four-year-old sections of the peony root that are typically used for their medicinal properties and mostly consumed in herbal teas or as a powdered supplement. However, peonies may live much, much longer—nobody knows for sure. What we do know is that they can outlive a human being and make it to one-hundred-plus years of age!

Herbalists and Traditional Chinese Medicine practitioners utilize white peony root for its ability to build and cleanse the blood, and to renew moisture to create flawless, radiant skin. The cleaner and healthier the blood, the more ageless we become! Peony's skin-enhancing properties don't end there. It also has mild antioxidant and antibacterial properties, which clear the skin of any inflammation or blemishes, creating that coveted youthful, radiant glow. Furthermore, as white peony root fortifies the blood, it acts to soothe and reduce inflammation throughout the body. This superherb also calms the mind, reduces stress, and induces sleep.

White peony's blood-supportive properties also make it a highly regarded women's herb for regulating the menstrual cycle and reducing cramping by relaxing the muscles. For centuries women have sworn by its hormone-regulating effects. When hormones don't yo-yo up and down throughout the month, women aren't affected by mood swings, acne, bloating, and back pain. Stable hormones are imperative to maintaining a beautiful visage.

CONCLUSION

I know you have been given a lot of information in this chapter—I tell people to be *under*whelmed, not overwhelmed. The important thing to remember is that just adding a few of these superfoods and super-herbs into your diet will really make a difference in how you look and feel. Check out what I typically eat in a day and you will see that I keep it pretty simple.

When I wake up: charcoal, enzymes, and sometimes silica supple-ments with pure spring water with a pinch of sea salt and honey. If I am in Hawaii, then I add a chunk of citrus fruit from my garden and/ or fresh noni juice. After about an hour I have a Nutriblast such as the Super Green Juice Nutriblast (page 247).

I drink lots of fresh spring water throughout the day or reishi and chaga mushroom iced tea, nettle tea, or horsetail tea. I am a tea drinker—it's a great way to stay hydrated and change things up!

Snack: my favorite? You guessed it: avocado with sea salt! And some-times I'll turn it into a small meal with some cruciferous veggies in a lettuce wrap or berries, which are in season in Canada as I write this book (blueberries, raspberries, blackberries, gooseberries, black cherries).

Lunch: leafy veggies from my garden—whatever is in season. For example, I just picked fresh nettle leaves. I also have a stir-fry of in-season veggies, cooked only briefly in coconut oil, drizzled with olive oil, and sprinkled with a little bit of sea salt.

Dinner: a taro or sweet potato, again drizzled with olive oil and sprin-kled with a pinch of sea salt, or an ancient grain like quinoa with a rainbow salad loaded with whatever vegetables I have harvested from my garden and/or the local farmers' market.

Dessert: a few cacao beans dipped in honey from my bee sanctuary.

As a nightcap before bed: reishi and chaga mushroom hot tea or sometimes a hot chocolate made with reishi and chaga tea blended with superfoods, plus a little chia seed or almond butter to give some "body" to the beverage.

Remove Toxins

Charles Dickens was right: we live in both the best of times *and* the worst of times. On the one hand, we have unprecedented access to extraordinary tools for beauty, health, and healing that can add more years to our life and more life to our years, enabling us to look and feel terrific at any age. On the other hand, we are constantly exposed to an onslaught of toxins in the air we breathe, the food we eat, the clothes we wear, the commercial beauty products we slather all over ourselves, and the water we drink.

The toll all of this takes on our physical, mental, and emotional health should not be underestimated. When our bodies lack the vitamins, minerals, enzymes, and oxygen they need to function optimally, our organs become overburdened with toxins and waste products, compromising the natural systems that escort these things from the body. Our internal organs, skin, hair, and nails are adversely affected. We age. We gain weight. Our skin loses its elasticity. We feel fatigued. We lack energy. We lose our spark.

The only thing more important for beauty than nutrition is detoxification. Which is exactly why removing toxins is the next beauty factor we need to discuss. When the body is loaded with toxins, even if we are choosing the best foods, we can't process or assimilate the nutrition effectively because our systems are too overworked. The answer: proper detoxification.

DETOXIFICATION: AN ANCIENT PRACTICE

Detoxification has a long history as a way to reset both the body and the mind to maximize health and longevity. Its recorded history began about three thousand years ago with ancient Egyptian and Greek civilizations, who promoted the act of flushing out the colon along with the practice of fasting to restore cellular health. Practitioners of the ancient Ayurvedic medicine system recommended plant-based elimination diets to regularly cleanse the body due to the belief that toxins accumulating in the digestive tract were the root cause of disease. Detoxification with herbs, and with the help of acupuncture and acupressure, was also a common practice in ancient Chinese tonic herbalism. Detox was looked at through the lens of energy flow and how to best support each organ to reduce stagnation. Indigenous tribes, including Native Americans, used herbs, sweating, and fasting to cleanse and purify on every level—mental, physical, and emotional.

These practitioners understood and emphasized detoxification, and they didn't live in a world nearly as overwhelmingly toxic as ours. There are millions of synthetic materials around us as well as a vast number of pesticides and herbicides, and even more toxic substances have been spilled into and polluted our waterways and airways. Our bodies are equipped to metabolize a certain amount of toxicity, but not the innumerable amount we are now exposed to as part of modern life.

Detoxification is all about arming the body with tools found in nature while removing all the built-up waste inside. When we wake up with dark circles under our eyes, have constant breakouts on our skin, or experience bloating, these are the warning signs that our bodies need us to change what we are eating, drinking, breathing, and even thinking!

We need to take a long-term approach to supporting the body and its incredible ability to self-heal, self-regulate, and thrive by aiding it in its natural detoxification processes. *When nature provides such exquisite and effective botanicals that graciously attend to our health and beauty, why use anything artificial?* In this way we can experience optimal health while also enjoying glowing skin, shiny hair, sparkling eyes, and strong teeth. We all need to "clean up our act" and optimize our ability to experience abundant health and radiant beauty.

Relying on the wisdom of our ancestors, I have put together a modern detoxification strategy so we all can enjoy abundant health, beauty, and youthfulness.

THE PATHWAYS OF DETOXIFICATION

Remember, beauty is from the *inside out*; therefore it begins with our internal organs. To create an outward appearance of beauty, we must maximize and support all our detoxification pathways. This includes the digestive and elimination system, liver, kidneys, lungs, skin, and lymphatic system. This chapter provides specific details on how best to detox and support each pathway in the body.

DIGESTIVE AND ELIMINATION SYSTEM

While digestion and elimination aren't necessarily the prettiest processes, if you don't address them, you can end up gassy, bloated, constipated, or with loose stools, which isn't very glamorous either.

Did you know that 70 percent of the body's immune system is in the digestive system? Improving your digestive system is one of the most beneficial ways to improve your overall health.

When your digestion is poor, your skin also suffers and you experience wrinkles, acne, eczema, blemishes, rosacea, rashes, and a dull complexion. Again, not so gorgeous.

Digestion begins with the mechanical digestion of food in the mouth and transitions into a chemical phase as food moves through the stomach and intestines. Food that can't be absorbed gets passed along through the body's sewer system and out of the body through the process of elimination.

Ideally, on its journey through the digestive system, food will be broken down into small enough compounds to be absorbed into the bloodstream as vital carbohydrates, proteins, fats, and vitamins to feed the cells so they can nourish the body. Unfortunately, the average American is on a diet of highly processed foods and harmful toxins, which impedes the body's ability to effectively absorb and assimilate minerals and vitamins during food's voyage through the thirty feet of digestive tract.

So let's dig into each part of the digestive process so we can understand it better and learn how to best support each step of the way for radiant beauty.

Step 1: Mouth

Chew your food at least twenty times before you swallow, David.

—MY MOM

Every night when I was little, my mom used to tell me to slow down and chew my food. It drove me crazy, because all I wanted to do was run back outside before it got dark, but her voice stuck in my head as I got older (as moms' voices tend to do). When I started studying digestion and nutrition, I realized once again that my mom was right!

Have you ever heard the expression "Your stomach can't chew food"? Proper digestion begins with the physical process of chewing. As you chew, your food breaks down into smaller and smaller particles and becomes partially liquefied, which makes it easier to digest and metabolize.

Chewing causes your mouth to secrete saliva, which coats your food with amylase and lipase, two important enzymes that digest fats and starches in your mouth. Chewing also cues the rest of the digestive tract to get ready to do its job—the stomach starts to prepare hydrochloric acid and the pancreas prepares to secrete its contents into the small intestinal tract. Research shows that it takes about twenty minutes for your brain to signal your stomach that you are full. The slower you eat, the less likely you are going to overeat, which can help avoid weight gain.

"Fight-or-flight eating" is what I call a new phenomenon developing in the Western world. We are so busy and stressed that eating "on the go" created a boom in fast-food chains at the cost of our health. When we stop chewing our food and quickly shovel it down the throat, we flood the body with cortisol, the fat-storing hormone. The digestive system has not adapted to this new way of eating, and the price we pay is ill-prepared and poorly digested meals. Eating in a stressed state is a quick way to pack on the pounds, and all this begins with the mind and the mouth.

People often attribute the slim waistlines of most Europeans to the Mediterranean diet. I would add that *the way they eat* is also very conducive to burning fat instead of storing it. They have a strong tradition of eating homemade meals with family and friends and taking well over an hour (sometimes three!) to enjoy their meals with some good company and conversation. Feeling connected with others and eating slowly maximizes the release of hormones, increases blood flow, satisfies appetite (reducing unhealthy food cravings), and encourages nutrient absorption.

In order to eat mindfully, put away your computer and cell phone, and have a quiet sit-down meal twice a day for twenty-five to forty-five minutes. Before you begin eating, take a moment to appreciate your meal. If you are stressed out, take two minutes to do a quiet breathing meditation. Remember to chew your food twenty to thirty times before swallowing it. Take your time, and relish each bite, without rushing or mindlessly shoving food into your mouth. Putting your fork down between mouthfuls is another strategy that helps slow down eating and prevent overeating. Eat until you feel satisfied but not stuffed. Try to plan a few meals a week with family and friends, and enjoy the company as much as the meal!

Step 2: Stomach

After chewing, you swallow, and the food travels down the esophagus into the stomach. You may feel happy and full, but the fun chemical part of the digestive process is only just ramping up inside.

In order to break down food, the stomach produces 3 liters of industrial-grade, super-concentrated hydrochloric acid each day, which packs enough power to chew through metal and bone. (Luckily the stomach also produces very large quantities of mucus to coat itself, so it remains unscathed by the corrosive HCL.) You need high levels of HCL to properly digest food. It's a myth that too much stomach acid is what causes heartburn. Too little HCL forces your stomach to churn and squeeze more to break down the food, which leaves the food in the stomach longer, causing gas and bloating. The gas and bloating put pressure on the esophagus, which can push it open, letting the HCL splash up into it, creating heartburn.

Here is a simple test you can do to determine the HCL level in your body: Look at your fingernails. If your cuticles are large and crescent-moon shaped, then you have a good amount of HCL. If they are very small or barely visible, you have low levels of HCL and you may need supplementation.

To help your stomach do its job optimally, you can

- Chew your food well so your stomach has more time to get the HCL brewing (I'm talking about the mom-recommended twenty or so chews mentioned previously).

- Add freshly squeezed lemon juice to water and drink it in between meals.

- Drink 1 to 2 teaspoons of raw apple cider vinegar in a glass of water before you eat.

Step 3: Small Intestine

From mouth to anus, your digestive system is about thirty feet long with twenty feet of it being your small intestine. That's a huge part of the digestive area in one system. Luckily for the muscles of the small intestine, it has the liver, pancreas, and gallbladder on its team to add digestive juices, further breaking down your food into absorbable particles. The walls of the small intestine then absorb the digested nutrients into the bloodstream. The blood delivers the nutrients to the rest of the body, and the magic of feeding your cells happens!

When it comes to the small intestine, absorption is key. One of the best ways to support the small intestine is to incorporate demulcents and fat into your diet. Demulcents soothe, hydrate, and heal the mucous membrane inside your intestines and protect against irritation and inflammation. Aloe vera gel tops the list. It's known to decrease the irritation and inflammation of irritable bowel syndrome (IBS), colitis, and other inflammatory disorders. More great demulcents

---

GMO Wheat Is the Worst

I highly recommend eliminating GMO wheat from your diet entirely. The semi-dwarf strain of wheat produced in America is a product of mutagenesis—washing the seed with chemicals to create a new strain of wheat that grows fast and short and can be harvested quickly. Although this is great for crop reports and the stock market, it is devastating for your digestion. Even if you show no symptoms of common disorders such as celiac disease and irritable bowel syndrome, your body is still working very hard to break down this entirely new class of food—and at the very least is producing an inflammatory response (more on this in "Balance Hormones," page 183). The wheat your great-grandparents ate is as different from modern wheat as apples are from oranges, for all practical purposes. For more detailed information on this subject, I recommend reading my friend Dr. William Davis's book *Wheat Belly.*

---

are chia seeds, slippery elm, licorice root, and Irish moss. An easy way to use these is to add them to your favorite smoothie. If you suffer from intestinal or bowel irritation, then a demulcent-rich diet is your top priority. (Check out the Eliminator recipe on page 108 for a drink that features natural demulcents.)

Another of my favorite tricks for nutrient absorption is to mix a small amount of oil into a blended vegetable drink or a veggie soup. Many of the oil-soluble vitamins, like A, E, and K, plus the key pigments found in vegetables are absorbed more readily in the presence of a small amount of heat and oil. Adding a teaspoon of olive oil or coconut oil to a blended drink is definitely an absorption hack and one that I use frequently. Adding oil to a salad is an age-old example of maximizing nutrient absorption. A study conducted by Purdue University and published in *Molecular Nutrition and Food Research* showed that eating low-fat or no-fat salad dressings resulted in fewer nutrients, like carotenoids, absorbed than when salads were eaten with full-fat dressings.

Step 4: Colon

After your body has absorbed everything it can through the walls of the small intestine, the remaining mixture moves into the large intestine, otherwise known as the colon. The colon's job is to absorb water from and compact what is left of your food as it moves forward. Billions of bacteria line the walls of the colon to help with the breakdown of the remaining organic matter. The continuous muscular action of the intestines transports this material through the body and ideally expels all of it, via the rectum, as stool.

Unfortunately, for millions of people, this ideal process does not occur. I have spoken to so many people over the years who ask me about gas, bloating, constipation, and acne. These are some of the most common complaints I hear. This is because if we're not eating a healthy, well-balanced diet, over time, feces can stop moving through the system quickly and start to build up on the intestinal walls. The backed-up poop accumulates harmful bacteria, which produce toxins. This then causes an inflammatory response, which slows things down even more. It's a cyclical problem that builds and builds.

Insufficient detoxification is devastating to the complexion. It sends toxins back into the body, where they eventually get pushed out of the skin as acne or rashes. If the colon is sluggish, then nutrient absorption by the rest of the digestive system will also be sluggish, making it hard to nourish the skin, hair, and nails. A gunked-up colon can also lead to more serious health situations as it becomes more impacted, and chronic inflammation sets in.

Think about this: The colon is roughly as long as you are tall—on average, five to six feet long. It is about as wide as your wrist and has the capacity to store between five and ten pounds of feces within each foot. This means you may easily have twenty-five to thirty pounds of waste stuck in your colon at any given time, especially if you eat a lot of meat.

Constipation is the number one sign that your colon is not moving waste out of your body rapidly enough to prevent inflammation. If you are not having three to four bowel movements a day, your body is not efficiently eliminating.

The first step is to add more fiber to your diet and drink more spring water. If you've done that and you're still not moving your bowels more than once a day, it may be time to consider colon hydrotherapy, in which a certified colon hydrotherapist will gently infuse your colon with warm water, stimulating the removal of gas, mucus, and encrusted fecal matter that has been there for weeks, months, or years.

You can also support your colon through the following Salt Water

---

The Second Brain

Recent discoveries show that a network of neurons lines our intestines, and it is brimming with neurotransmitters. This network runs from the esophagus to the anus and contains approximately 100 million neurons, more than in the peripheral nervous system or the spinal cord.

Technically known as the enteric nervous system, this "second brain" is embedded in the walls of the gut and allows us to "feel" the inner world of our long gut and its contents. The second brain informs our state of mind in other ways as well: 95 percent of the body's serotonin is found in the second brain. This means our emotions and mental state can have a powerful effect on our digestion. Stress can quickly shut down the digestive processes. The simplest thought by the brain can produce immediate chemical reactions in the gut— for good or for bad.

Flush, a home remedy to help with detoxification. As the salt moves through your digestive system, beginning in the mouth, it will activate the enzymes needed to break down your food on its way to the stomach. In the stomach, it will promote the formation of hydrochloric acid. As it travels farther, the mineralized salt will act upon your hormones—your metabolic processes involving the breakdown of proteins and glucose—and will harmonize with other minerals to balance the pH in your body. Once it reaches your colon, the extra fluid and sea salt will work together to scrub the walls of your colon, forcing the excretion of built-up fecal matter and the toxins that cling to it.

Salt Water Flush

1 to 2 tablespoons freshly squeezed lime or lemon juice

8 to 10 ounces spring water, gently heated (keep below 110°F so as not to destroy the enzymes in the citrus juice)

2 teaspoons sea salt (which will *not* be totally white if it is true sea salt!)

Stir all the ingredients together in a glass jar until the salt dissolves, then drink it quickly, downing it within 5 minutes. This is best done first thing in the morning on an empty stomach, but it can be done at any time throughout the day as long as you have not eaten within the past few hours, and make sure you have no plans for several hours afterward—unless they involve easy access to a toilet!

Remember, not only are you lightening up your toxic load and shedding the sluggishness that comes from an overburdened colon; you're also flooding your intestines with the soothing properties of sea salt.

The same sea salt that soothes aching muscles and reduces inflammation when used topically is going to help soothe the inflammation in your gut when ingested.

Step 5: Elimination

Your bathroom behavior provides important clues about your digestive health. How often you go, how long it takes, what it looks like all matter. It is critical to have regular bowel movements; if you do not, debris builds up in your body, which is not good for your health or your beauty. Try the following drink for optimal digestion and elimination.

The Eliminator

This hydrating elixir provides abundant fiber, important electrolytes, natural demulcents, probiotics, and herbs—all key ingredients for maintaining healthy digestive balance and regularity. A healthy colon is directly related to clear, beautiful, lustrous skin.

16 ounces spring water

4-inch piece fresh aloe vera, skin removed

1 lemon, peeled

½ to 1 cup fresh or frozen berries (your favorite kind)

1 tablespoon chia seeds

½ teaspoon probiotic powder (adjust the amount according to your tolerance)

½ teaspoon camu or amla berry powder

½-inch piece fresh ginger root

Pinch of sea salt

Raw organic honey or stevia to taste

Blend all the ingredients together in a high-speed blender and enjoy. This elixir may be used as a meal replacement—it's filling and tastes amazing!

Note: Intestinal issues are often caused by a bacterial imbalance, so if you know you have candida or blood sugar issues, it would be best to use stevia rather than honey. If you do not have issues regarding sugar, raw honey adds additional nutritional benefits.

LIVER

Weighing in at three hefty pounds, the liver is one of our hardest working organs and sits in rank as the second largest, after the skin. The liver performs more than five hundred vital functions (many of these simultaneously!) with its two primary goals being digestion and detoxification.

The liver is the metabolic beauty factory of the body. It stores sugar, and whenever the cells need energy, the liver provides it by converting this storage into energy. It sustains all the functions performed every minute by the body's cells to keep us youthful and radiant. The heart depends on energy from the liver, and it pumps nutrient rich blood to the skin, maintaining collagen production and oxygenating the cells to protect against premature aging. The hair follicles need energy sent to them in order to grow shiny, lustrous locks. The nails need energy to grow smooth and strong without ridges or dents.

By processing a liter or more of blood per minute, the liver breaks down all the nutrients leaving the stomach and intestines into forms the rest of the body can use effectively. It uses these nutrients to manufacture its own proteins, regulate hormones (like estrogen and testosterone), process fats, store sugars, produce enzymes to clot the blood, and detoxify the body.

The liver functions as a filter for everything we are exposed to in the air we breathe, the food we eat, the water we drink, and what we put on and in the body. It is the liver's job to filter and get rid of anything harmful or toxic to keep the body healthy and strong. This critical beauty organ is so important that when it stops functioning we can't survive.

A hundred years ago, the liver didn't have to worry about too much external toxicity and liver disease was rare. In today's world, the liver is under constant siege by processed foods, excess sugars, rancid fats, environmental toxins, and a lack of proper hydration.

Spots on the skin and in the eyes as well as puffiness around the eyes are indications of an underperforming liver. If your liver is not doing its job of breaking down toxins efficiently, the toxins need to be eliminated through your skin. Excessive toxin buildup causes inflammation, which can manifest as eczema, dermatitis, wrinkles, brown liver spots, red itchy rashes, hives, psoriasis, rosacea, or acne.

Five Flavor Detox Salad

This incredible detox salad feeds all your organ systems and supports healthy cleansing.

For the salad

> **Mixed greens (baby kale, romaine, spinach, etc.)**
> **1 pint fresh blueberries**
> **½ cup shredded or diced, cooked or fermented beet**
> **½ cucumber, diced**
> **2 stalks celery, chopped**
> **6 to 12 chlorella tablets**
> **1 avocado, diced (optional)**

For the dressing

- ¼ cup olive oil
- 2 ounces spring water
- ¼ cup raw pumpkin seeds
- 1 clove garlic
- ½-inch piece fresh ginger root or ¼ teaspoon ground ginger
- Handful of freshly chopped parsley or cilantro
- 3 tablespoons freshly squeezed lemon juice
- 1 tablespoon apple cider vinegar
- Pinch of Celtic or Icelandic sea salt

Rinse and chop greens into bite-size pieces and place the greens in a large salad bowl. Add the blueberries, beet, cucumber, and celery. Set the bowl aside.

To make the dressing, place all the dressing ingredients in a high-speed blender or food processor and blend the mixture until it is creamy. (Alternatively, you can add the pumpkin seeds separately to the salad after soaking to soften them.) Adjust the dressing to taste.

Drizzle the salad with the dressing, and add the chlorella tablets and the optional avocado right before serving. The combination of the salad and the dressing covers all five flavors: sweet, sour, salty, bitter, and pungent (umami).

In the pursuit of beauty and well-being, we must be proactive about supporting the liver. This means removing the burdens the liver carries and then aiding it with superfood and superherb nutrition. In this way we can stabilize our hormones, purify our blood, deliver nutrients to our skin, and keep energy flowing throughout our body.

Liver Detoxification

The liver handles toxins in a two-step process known as phase I and phase II liver detoxification. The liver not only has to break down and eliminate toxins that arise from normal metabolic functions but also must contend with the thousands of chemicals being dumped into the environment these days—many of which are classified as endocrine disruptors and affect hormones in staggering ways.

When the liver is overtaxed and sluggish, it can't counteract the devastating effects these human-made chemicals have on our health and appearance, so it's critically important to support the liver in its detoxification.

In *phase I* of liver detoxification, enzymes are released to oxidize and reduce toxins into smaller, water-soluble forms more easily eliminated by the body. Most of the dangerous toxins we are exposed to are fat-soluble and must be broken down in order to be eliminated through urine, excrement, or sweating. If we don't support phase I detoxification, these fat-soluble toxins will find their way into our fat cells, where they fester for long periods of time.

Breaking down toxins produces free radicals, which are very damaging to the body. To neutralize free radicals, the liver uses its own antioxidants—primarily glutathione, one of the body's most important antioxidants, without which the liver would damage itself in the process of detoxification. The body can recycle and reuse glutathione, but when there is a toxic overload, this delicate system is thrown out of balance and can enter a downward spiral, taking our beauty and health along with it.

In *phase II*, the liver adds chemicals to the broken-down toxins to make them safe for removal. This is called "conjugation" and is the final step before elimination. The body's ability to methylate properly is vitally important at this stage, although methylation is critical for every cell in the body to function. It controls the replication of DNA and the aging process of each individual cell. Methyl groups come from fresh fruits and vegetables, especially dark leafy greens, as well as other sulfur-containing foods. Reducing alcohol and excess sugar helps with methylation, as does the supplement methylsulfonylmethane. Once the toxins are made water-soluble and packaged for elimination, they will exit the body.

Make yourself aware of the symptoms of liver dysfunction, included in the following list. If you suspect your liver is not detoxifying properly, limit the items that cause an imbalance and/or dysfunction and add into your diet some of the supplements and herbs that will support your liver. I've also included next a terrific drink, called the Liver Regenerator.

Symptoms of liver dysfunction: acne, constant bloating, eczema, hives, liver spots, psoriasis, rashes, rosacea, wrinkles, yellow skin and/or eyes (sign of jaundice).

Causes of liver imbalance or dysfunction: anger, conventionally grown fruits and vegetables, factory-farmed meat and dairy, high alcohol intake, high-fructose corn syrup, hormonal imbalances, poor diet, refined sugars, sedentary lifestyle, stress.

Liver-supporting plants and herbs: bupleurum, burdock root, cardamom, cilantro, coconut oil, dandelion root, green tea, holy basil (tulsi), hot water with lemon first thing in the morning, milk thistle, parsley, schizandra, turmeric.

The Liver Regenerator

12 ounces nut milk

1 tablespoon coconut oil, melted

2 teaspoons MSM powder

½ teaspoon ground turmeric

¼ teaspoon ground cinnamon
Dash of black pepper
Raw organic honey or stevia to taste

Heat the nut milk in a saucepan until it starts to bubble but not boil. Add the warm nut milk to a high-speed blender with all the remaining ingredients—the coconut oil, MSM, turmeric, cinnamon, black pepper, and sweetener—and blend the mixture until it's frothy. Adjust the sweetener to taste. Enjoy this regenerator before bed for a great night's sleep!

My preferred nondairy milk is coconut milk. It's rich and creamy, and it gives a great texture to any drink (like the Liver Regenerator), plus it has healthy medium-chain fatty acids that are easily converted to energy. If you prefer to choose a different kind of nondairy milk, homemade nut milks are ideal whenever possible. The best nuts for liver health are the ones that are well protected from pesticides and environmental toxins because of their shells, including almonds, Brazil nuts, pecans, and walnuts. Always try to buy organic, raw nuts—not roasted.

Turmeric contains antioxidant and anti-inflammatory properties. It is a great support for a healthy liver and is best absorbed when taken in combination with a fat (like coconut oil) and with black pepper, which enhances its bioavailability.

KIDNEYS

In Traditional Chinese Medicine, the two bean-shaped kidneys that flank the spine are considered the most important organs from a longevity point of view and are critical in maintaining beauty and radiance. They keep the composition of the blood stable by preventing extra waste and fluid from building up while also maintaining the electrolyte balance needed for healthy nerve function. They are the body's filtration system too. They process blood and are key in keeping the skin hydrated and the blood clean. They remove the waste products of protein metabolism, like ammonia, nitrogen, and uric acid, as well as other toxins, such as drugs, excess hormones, food additives, minerals, and vitamins. Every twenty-four hours they filter about two hundred quarts of blood and make about one to two quarts of urine!

The kidneys make a hormone called erythropoietin, which prompts bone marrow to make red blood cells. Red blood cells carry oxygen from the lungs to supply all the body's beauty needs. They provide the energy needed to grow strong nails and give skin a healthy glow. When the blood is weak, it can't feed the bones and nourish the hair, and you end up with brittle bones and hair loss.

The kidneys are involved in regulating the amount of water in the body. When you consume too much liquid, the kidneys increase urination. When you drink too little, they retain water. Water maintains the moisture content of the skin at a high level, keeping it plump and dewy looking. Because the kidneys regulate water metabolism, puffiness under the eyes can be the result of kidney dysfunction. Water retention and bloating are also connected to improperly functioning kidneys.

When you use commercial beauty products that contain phthalates, hydroquinone, parabens, and a slew of other toxic chemicals, these enter your bloodstream and have to pass through your kidneys. Commercial beauty products also contain heavy metals, including lead, arsenic, mercury, and aluminum, which are micronized for commercial use. These small particles need to be filtered by your kidneys too. If you slather these products on your body every single day, eventually your kidneys will be unable to keep up.

As the kidneys become overloaded with these dangerous chemicals and harmful toxins, dark circles can appear under your eyes, you can have trouble sleeping, or you can feel fatigued. If you are already experiencing these signs, then it is crucial you take immediate action. The kidneys are your jing organs, so jing herbs—like he shou wu and others—should be consumed daily (see "Superfoods and Superherbs," beginning on page 49).

My favorite way to take good care of my kidneys is through spring water nutrition. Maintaining proper hydration with clean, pure spring water gives kidney health a massive upgrade. Most people are dehydrated, and when they do drink water, it is municipal tap water, polluted with heavy metals and industrial chemicals. I am a wild spring water hunter. There is nothing like drinking fresh spring water. It is extremely invigorating, and the intangible benefits will probably not be properly measured by science within our lifetimes. When we bestow spring water upon our kidneys, we infuse them with the charge placed on the water over thousands of years by the earth's filtration. See "Cellular Hydration" on page 167 to learn more about the benefits of spring water and how to stay properly hydrated.

LUNGS

The lungs are a central part of the respiratory system, the group of organs and tissues that work together to help you breathe. The lungs' main function is to transport oxygen from the atmosphere into the body when you inhale and to release carbon dioxide from the body when you exhale. Every cell in the body needs oxygen in order to live, so the process of breathing is critical to a healthy, beautiful existence.

Each one of your cells needs a steady supply of oxygen to produce energy. Without oxygen, cellular function becomes impaired and cell death or damage occurs. Once oxygen enters the lungs, it's moved into the bloodstream and carried throughout the body to fuel the cells. As the cells create energy, they release waste products, one of which is carbon dioxide. The bloodstream carries this waste gas back to the lungs, where it is removed from the bloodstream and then exhaled.

Hair thrives with a rich supply of oxygenated, nutrient-rich blood pumping to its follicles. Proper blood circulation to the scalp encourages steady hair growth and thickness. Lack of oxygen and other nutrients causes brittle, dull, thin hair, so maintaining the health of your lungs is vital to your lovely locks.

The circulation of oxygen-rich blood from the lungs provides the skin with deep nourishment as well. Oxygen stimulates collagen and elastin production, and helps to maintain the structural integrity of the skin by boosting circulation and stimulating cell turnover, leaving your complexion hydrated and revitalized. The opening and closing of the skin's pores are also governed by the lungs, allowing the skin to clear toxins that may be stuck there.

High concentrations of oxygen are also anti-inflammatory and trigger the body's natural healing functions. In an oxygen-rich environment, bacteria, viruses, and fungal infections simply do not survive, thus the lungs support the immune system in keeping the body strong and supple.

Interestingly, in Traditional Chinese Medicine the lungs, spleen, skin, and colon are considered closely connected. The skin is called the "outer lung," and it is responsible for the first level of immunity. Scientifically speaking, the skin cannot absorb oxygen like the lungs, but from a TCM energy point of view, it absorbs substances from the environment and expels toxins from inside, just as the lungs do, making them similar in function. If this mechanism is broken due to weak lung capacity or poor function, then the skin begins to dry up and its luster fades.

Since the lungs are always working, even while you sleep, it is important to keep them healthy. A great way to increase your lung capacity is through swimming, which is something I do every day when I am in Hawaii. You might also have a delicious drink with magnificent lung-supporting ingredients, like this one:

Love Your Lungs Tonic

2 cups gynostemma tea, warm

1 tablespoon coconut oil

1 tablespoon lucuma powder

1 teaspoon chaga powder

1 teaspoon astragalus powder

1 teaspoon cordyceps powder

¼ teaspoon vanilla powder

Raw organic honey to taste

Blend all the ingredients together in a high-speed blender and enjoy!

SKIN

The surface of our skin is teeming with billions of tiny bacteria that manage our health and communicate with and educate our internal immune system. Our amazing skin protects us against UV radiation, pathogens, viruses, harmful bacteria, parasites, dehydration, and infection. Everything we put on our skin directly affects this delicate layer of bacteria and will determine the skin's health, look, and feel. Skin flora that is wiped out by repeated use of antibiotic creams and synthetic cosmetics leaves us wide open to an array of skin irritations and even skin disease.

We need to think of our skin as an intricate and bustling ecosystem of living organisms instead of a piece of drywall in need of a coat of paint. Only by realizing this can we break out of the vicious cycle of covering and masking our skin problems with skin-flora-killing products, leading to even more use of commercial cosmetics.

The integumentary system (a fancy name for the skin) is also a passageway that gets rid of toxins in the body and protects us from the harmful buildup of cellular waste material. Every minute we shed 30,000 to 40,000 dead skin cells—that's nearly 9 pounds a year!

Here are some more interesting facts about skin:

- The average person has about 300 million skin cells.

- A single square inch of skin has about 19 million cells and up to 300 sweat glands.

- Your skin accounts for 15 percent of your body weight.

- Your skin is thickest on your feet (1.4 millimeters) and thinnest on your eyelids (0.2 millimeters).

- Your skin renews itself every 28 days.

- The average person's skin covers an area of 2 square meters and contains more than 11 miles of blood vessels.

From a detoxification point of view, it is imperative to have open and clear pores. One of the biggest challenges that arise from using commercial beauty products is their inherent tendency to block pores and create stagnation. To clear the detoxification pathway of the skin, an obvious first step is to stop adding toxins to this pathway. Also, the delicate skin of infants and young children is estimated to be five times thinner than the skin of adults and can therefore absorb substances far more easily, so it's extra important to think about what we're slathering on our kids.

Let's take a look at some of the worst beauty offenders in commercial beauty products.

TOXINS IN COMMERCIAL BEAUTY PRODUCTS

There are countless toxic ingredients added into commercial skin care products—I could write an entire book on the subject and some people have. Read *Not Just a Pretty Face: The Ugly Side of the Beauty Industry* by Stacy Malkan for more information. I highly recommend educating yourself more on this topic by referring to the Environmental Working Group Skin Deep Cosmetics Database (ewg.org/skindeep/), which is a phenomenal resource for toxic ingredients lurking in commercial beauty products. Health studies and pretesting are not required by the government for these products before they are sold, and only 200 of the 80,000 chemicals in this country have been tested for safety. Below are ten of the worst ingredients, but there are many, many more you should be aware of and avoid. Remember: your skin is highly permeable—which means what you put *on* your body is as important as what you put *in* it!

1. Artificial Colors and Dyes: Used to create alluring colors, the majority of these laboratory-created hues are derived from petroleum or coal tar sources and can be contaminated with things like benzidine and 4-aminobiphenyl, which are known human carcinogens. The European Commission's Classification, Labelling, and Packaging regulation considers all synthetic colors to be human carcinogens, but the FDA still allows seven to be used in the US. "D&C" preceding a color and number (e.g., D&C Red 27) on a label means "Drug and Cosmetic" artificial color. When it's followed by the word "lake," it indicates that the pigment is mixed with calcium or aluminum as a fixative so the color stays when applied to the skin; this is why certain lipsticks don't bleed.

Watch out for: conditioners; cosmetics such as blush, eye shadow, and lipstick; deodorants; hand soaps; lotions; nail polishes; shampoos; and toothpastes.

2. Dioxane: 1,4-Dioxane is a known eye and respiratory tract irritant that easily penetrates the skin. The National Toxicology Program has titled it a known animal carcinogen, and the Environmental Protection Agency has classified it as a probable human carcinogen (no human trials have been conducted). As a chemical solvent primarily used in the manufacturing process, dioxane is hidden in thousands of products. The only way to know that the product you use is free of dioxane is if it sports the USDA Organic certification seal.

Watch out for: anti-aging products, baby soaps, body firming lotions, body washes, bubble baths, hair dyes and bleaches, deodorants, eye serums, facial moisturizers, hair relaxers, mouthwashes, shampoos, sunless tanning products, and toothpastes.

3. Fragrances/Parfum, Synthetic: These words can indicate up to a thousand toxic and/or carcinogenic substances, including phthalates, which create the scent added to a product. According to the FDA and to the Environmental Working Group (EWG) Skin Deep Cosmetics Database, synthetic fragrances may cause allergies, headaches, dizziness, dermatitis, skin discoloration, skin irritation, violent coughing, vomiting, and potential effects on the reproductive system.

Watch out for: body washes, colognes/perfumes, conditioners, deodorants, moisturizers, sanitary pads, shampoos, and tampons.

4. Formaldehyde: Determined by the World Health Organization's International Agency for Research on Cancer (IARC) and the US Department of Health and Human Services to be a human carcinogen, formaldehyde is used to prevent bacterial growth in cosmetic products. This preservative has been linked to nasal and nasopharyngeal cancers, can cause unsightly skin reactions, and can be harmful to the immune system. Also, keep an eye out for the following chemicals, which react with water within the product's bottle to create formaldehyde: DMDM hydantoin, imidazolidinyl urea, diazolidinyl urea, and quaternium-15.

Watch out for: body washes for adults and children, bubble baths, conditioners, eye shadows, hair straighteners, nail polishes, and shampoos.

5. Polyethylene Glycol (PEG): Ethylene compounds are nervous system depressants and potentially toxic to the liver and kidneys. PEG in and of itself is not a major concern, however it is generally contaminated with dioxane (see description above), ethylene oxide, and heavy metals, which are known to cause kidney, neurological, and autoimmune issues. Manufacturers could spend the money to strip these toxins out but most often leave them in to cut costs; therefore it's best to avoid all products containing ethylenes.

Watch out for: antimicrobial creams, cosmetics, conditioners, deodorants, moisturizers, sanitary pads, shampoos, and tampons.

6. Sodium Benzoate: This very common preservative is found at the end of many ingredient lists. While on its own it may seem innocuous, when it comes into contact with citric acid or ascorbic acid (vitamin C)—whether in the rest of the ingredients or present in your body—it morphs into a known carcinogen called benzene. It's worthwhile to note that sodium benzoate is often used to preserve extracts and so it may be hidden within an ingredient. For example, while "calendula officinalis extract" may be listed as an ingredient on the label, it could be preserved with sodium benzoate.

Watch out for: conditioners, cosmetics, deodorants, hand soaps, lotions, mouthwashes, shampoos, skin care products, and toothpastes.

7. Sulfates: Ninety percent of foaming and lathering products contain sulfates. Sulfates are frequently described on labels as "comes from" or "derived from" coconut in an effort to portray them as natural, even though they are known skin and eye irritants and hormone and endocrine disruptors, create organ toxicity, are suspected carcinogens, and can cause labored breathing and diarrhea. Over 16,000 studies have been done on this chemical addressing a long list of concerns. On labels, avoid sodium laureth sulfate (SLES), ammonium laureth sulfate (ALES), sodium lauryl sulfate (SLS), and ammonium lauryl sulfate (ALS).

Watch out for: body washes, cosmetics, hair color and bleaching agents, hair spray, liquid hand soaps, mouthwashes, perfumes, powders, scalp treatments, shampoos, sunscreens, and toothpastes.

8. Urea: The American Academy of Dermatology reports that urea is a primary cause of contact dermatitis, especially in concentrated amounts found in skin exfoliants. It remains on the skin for hours, giving it plenty of time to absorb into your skin cells as it works to soften them. Urea's other job is to mix with parabens to create formaldehyde, a toxic preservative discussed above. On a label, you may see it written as diazolidinyl urea, imidazolidinyl urea, or DMDM hydantoin.

Watch out for: anti-aging treatments, cleansers, conditioners, deodorants, eye creams, face masks, foundations, hair dyes, lotions, mouthwashes, shampoos, shaving creams, styling gels, water-based cosmetics, and sunscreens.

9. Parabens: For a detailed description of the dangers of parabens, please see page 194.

10. Phthalates: These chemicals are so toxic they are worth mentioning here again. I delve into the details in the hormone chapter, so please reference page 194.

Final Thought

Remember that smearing chemicals on your skin is arguably even worse than eating them because they move directly into the bloodstream. When toxins enter through your digestive system, they can be broken down and filtered first, reducing their impact. The Environmental Working Group estimates that one out of five cosmetics could contain a cancer-causing substance. Do you want that seeping directly into your blood?

Essential Oils

Essential oils are highly concentrated botanical extracts that contain valuable properties for beautifying your skin. They are natural, nontoxic, and packed with powerful antioxidants, which contribute to healthy, happy, hydrated smooth skin that glows! Essential oils are a really great natural alternative to commercial beauty products and have a tremendous history going back more than five thousand years. They have benefits ranging from beautifying the skin to wound healing to immune system support. Be warned: an oil labeled as an "extraction" is different from a "distillation"; in extracted essential oils, chemicals have been used to separate the plant's volatile aromatic compound (VAC), which is not considered ideal for health. I use only distilled essential oils.

All essential oils are antibacterial, antiviral, and antifungal. These compounds are what plants use to defend themselves against opportunistic organisms, like mold and fungus. The unique characteristic of many essential oils is the ability to kill harmful bacteria without killing beneficial bacteria. They have the innate intelligence of the plant and create an optimal environment for health and beauty, especially when used topically.

The phytochemicals found in plants have been developed over thousands of years. By harnessing their power we can heal and nourish our skin as well as lift our mood. When you use aromatherapy and essential oils on the skin, you are creating a healthy environment in which beneficial bacteria can easily grow. Whether our skin glows or not will depend largely upon the health of our skin's microbiome.

Essential oils also penetrate the blood–brain barrier and can easily pass through your cellular matrix. This means that when you use essential oils topically, they penetrate the various layers of skin and heal and nourish on a very deep level. Because they are natural "antibiotics" and do not kill the beneficial bacteria on the skin, only the harmful microorganisms, I have included them here in detoxification.

My good friend Nadine Artemis, an authority on beauty and essential oils and author of the incredible book *Renegade Beauty*, ranks here the top essential oils to use topically for optimal skin nutrition:

- chamomile
- frankincense
- immortelle
- lavender
- palmarosa
- peppermint
- rose otto
- sandalwood
- seabuckthorn berry
- sweet thyme

One way I get essential oils into my body is by taking a Detox Bath. This is my favorite way to bathe.

Detox Bath

¼ cup Icelandic flake salt

¼ cup Epsom salt

¼ cup baking soda

⅓ cup apple cider vinegar

10 drops of your favorite essential oil (I usually use Douglas fir, frankincense, immortelle, lavender, sandalwood, or a combination of these)

Combine the Icelandic flake salt, Epsom salt, and baking soda. Stir the combination into a quart of warm water until it dissolves.

Fill your bathtub, and add to it the apple cider vinegar and the desired essential oil. Pour in the dissolved salt mixture.

Soak in the bath for 30 to 60 minutes. Repeat this once a week. Also, make sure you drink extra water during the following 24 to 48 hours as your body continues to move unwanted toxins through your system.

LYMPHATIC SYSTEM

The lymphatic system supports the circulatory system by removing excess fluids and proteins from tissues and putting them back into the bloodstream. It also serves as a defense system for the body, filtering out disease-causing organisms, producing white blood cells, and generating antibodies. Without the lymphatic system, tissues would swell and the body would soon be overwhelmed by infection and toxicity.

A major part of the immune system, the lymphatic system is a network of organs that includes the spleen, lymph nodes, and lymph vessels. The lymph nodes house the white blood cells and act as a filter for toxins and opportunistic organisms, while the lymph vessels transport the lymph fluid throughout the body. This fluid is made up of white blood cells (lymphocytes) and interstitial fluid, which bathes cells and washes away unwanted toxins.

The lymphatic system moves in one direction only: upward. It is constantly resisting gravitational forces and is therefore a youth and longevity system.

All detoxification occurs first and foremost via the lymphatic system since the body contains more lymph fluid than blood. When you have poor blood circulation, the lymphatic system cannot properly do its job because toxins do not get removed from the body in a timely manner. This results in cellulite, varicose veins, and a weakened immune system. Also, because the lymphatic system removes infection, and acne is oftentimes an infection, a sluggish lymph system can be a secondary cause of acne.

As I mentioned, the skin is the largest eliminative organ of the body. It is a highly functioning and intelligent drainage system for the body. However, it is less than ideal to have toxins coming out through the skin; this is generally a sign that the other eliminative functions of the body are overburdened—like the lymphatic system. Because the lymphatic system runs just underneath the skin, it is imperative to keep it moving. When it becomes sluggish, this affects the quality of your skin. If you have ever popped a zit and seen clear fluid come out, that was lymph fluid. Most likely your lymph system was overworked or backed up, and the backup rose through your skin.

To develop and maintain beauty, you need to make sure you are not burdening the lymphatic system unnecessarily but rather making its job easier. Here are some of my favorite lymph-supporting activities:

Rebounding is the act of jumping lightly on a mini trampoline. It pumps the lymph and stimulates drainage. It also gives you an incredible workout with little or no chance of injury.

Dry brushing is a method of lymph stimulation that should be done less frequently—maybe once or twice a week—because over-exfoliation of the skin isn't helpful and can create more problems. (See "Dry Brushing" on page 130 for instructions.)

Yoga and tai chi use the subtle energy of the nervous system to stimulate lymph movement. Also, because breath is key to the lymph pump, yoga and tai chi improve the way we breathe. Deep breathing is essential for beauty and skin health because it moves the lymph and oxygenates the blood, bringing nutrients more easily to different skin layers.

Hot and cold therapy is an ancient technique that ramps up metabolism and strengthens the immune system. I have spent a lot of time in Iceland, and one of the first things I do there is alternate ice bathing in the ocean with sauna sitting. The contractions of the muscles during hot and cold therapy are perfect for pumping the lymph. A simple way to engage in hot and cold hydrotherapy each morning is to use hot and cold water in the shower. Combined with occasional cold

plunges and sauna time, this is extremely effective, increases circulation to the skin, and releases a hormonal cascade that makes you look
and feel younger!

As hydrotherapy and cryotherapy (cold therapy) are scientifically
studied for their anti-inflammatory properties, more benefits are
becoming known. As an added perk, even when you are submerged
in moderately cool water, neurotransmitters are released throughout
the body, specifically noradrenaline and dopamine. When you have a
surge in dopamine, guess what happens to your cortisol levels? That
hormone responsible for stress eating and unwanted belly fat goes
down! Also, your body goes into a rapid fat-burning state that can last
for hours.

All of these therapies show great promise for enhancing your personal
beauty.

TOXINS IN THE CLOTHES WE WEAR

- The skin is the largest and most porous organ in the body. Up to 64 percent
  of what we put on it is absorbed into the bloodstream—*some believe it is
  absorbed within just twenty-six seconds!*
- Clothing manufacturers use over eight thousand dangerous synthetic
  chemicals to produce the garments we wear, and the number of chemicals
  continues to grow every year.
- A 2015 Stockholm University analysis of sixty random garments from several
  international clothing chains revealed the presence of thousands of chemicals, many *not* revealed on the manufacturers' lists.
- Cotton is considered the world's "dirtiest" crop. It's responsible for the use of
  over 3.3 billion dollars' worth of chemical pesticides each year, half of which
  are considered toxic enough to be classified as highly hazardous by the
  World Health Organization.

- Even baby clothes made from organic cotton may legally contain dangerous chemicals like heavy metals and chlorine.
- Perfluorinated chemicals (PFCs), such as Teflon and Scotchgard, are known cancer-causing compounds, yet they are increasingly added to children's clothing, including compulsory school uniforms, because they add durability and make them wrinkle-, water-, and stain-resistant.
- The US places no restrictions on the use of formaldehyde or formaldehyde-releasing ingredients in clothing—linked to skin and lung irritation, headaches, contact dermatitis, and even cancer—while most other governments restrict or have banned its use entirely.

WHAT CAN WE DO ABOUT IT?

- Buy clothing made only of natural fibers, such as hemp. Hemp is sustainable, requires about half the amount of water cotton requires to grow, does not require pesticides, and is durable, breathable, and naturally water-resistant.
- Wash new clothes before wearing them. Washing may not remove *all* chemicals from clothing, but it can greatly reduce some of them, including formaldehyde resins.
- Stop buying so many new clothes. Buy used clothing to help cut down manufacturing demands and keep items out of landfills. Plus, clothing that has already been washed and worn several times will have already leached out many of the toxic chemicals.
- Look for safe-certified labels, such as the OEKO-TEX Standard 100 label, which confirms by an independent laboratory that the clothing is free of harmful levels of more than one hundred substances.
- Examine care instructions before buying clothing. Certain words and phrases, such as "permanent press," "durable," "stain resistant," "flame resistant," "wrinkle-free," and "easy care," are clear giveaways that the textile is toxic.

DETOXIFICATION METHODS

Regular and strategic detoxification is crucial for beauty. The following are my favorite ways to remove toxins naturally.

DRY BRUSHING

Dry brushing is a time-proven strategy to improve the skin and lymphatic system. Brushing the skin helps to stimulate lymph flow within the body, moving stuck toxins out of the connective tissues. It improves circulation, delivering oxygenated blood to the skin, which helps reduce the appearance of cellulite, wrinkles, and age spots. This results in a glowing complexion with an even skin tone and pores free of oil, dirt, and grime. Dry brushing also softens hard fat deposits below the skin while distributing them more evenly, promoting tighter skin and cell renewal.

Follow the directions I provide next for an invigorating dry brushing session, and remember while doing it that the pressure you apply should be firm, but not painful. Do not brush over broken skin (cuts, patches of eczema, etc.), sensitive areas, varicose veins, or bruises; and do not brush your face (unless you use a special brush made for this). Of course, dry brush when your body is *dry* (hence the name "dry brushing"). It's best to do right before you shower.

How to Dry Brush Your Body

- Purchase a natural bristle brush with a long handle so you can reach all areas of your body.
- Add a few drops of organic coconut oil to the bristles of your brush.
- Start on the sole of your right foot. (You may find it helpful to sit

down.) Brush up your ankle, shin, calf, and knee. Then do the same on your left side.

- Next, stand up (if you are sitting) and brush your right and then left thigh from the knee up. Be sure to get the inner thigh, which is a key spot for removing toxins.

- Move over to your abdomen, brushing in a counterclockwise motion.

- Brush each arm, starting with the palm, inward toward your heart. (Always brush toward your heart, because lymph flows toward the heart; brushing away from your heart can put pressure on your veins.) The armpit area is another area toxins like to accumulate, so make sure to pay close attention there.

- Gently brush the chest area, but not your actual breasts or nipples.

- Brush the neck area by starting at the nape of your neck and stroking over the shoulder to the front.

- Lastly, brush your back.

- Shake your brush over the sink or trash to get rid of skin cells. About once a week wash it with soap and water, then let it dry completely before using it again.

- Take a shower after you dry brush. Consider taking a contrast shower (alternating between the hottest water temperature you can stand and the coldest) to stimulate blood circulation and lymph drainage.

- After getting out of the shower, dry off and massage your skin with organic coconut oil or cacao butter.

Tip: After dry brushing, drink a glass of warm water with lemon. It hydrates the lymphatic system and supports a healthy body pH, detoxification, the elimination of toxins, and weight loss.

A word to the wise: skin pushes up new skin cells from underneath and needs the top layer of dead cells for a short period of time to serve as protection. This layer of dead cells also functions as food for the surface bacteria that inhabit the microbiome. I suggest dry brushing only when you feel you have a lot of skin cell pileup or you are dealing with a specific issue.

CLAY

Clay is an incredible substance that has been used for its ability to detoxify and heal the body both internally and externally. Aristotle made the first reference to humans deliberately ingesting clay and soil for health purposes; Marco Polo, in the description of his travels, shared how he saw Muslim pilgrims eat "pink earth" and cure themselves of fevers; Cleopatra used clay from the Nile River and the Arabian Desert as part of her elaborate beauty regimen; Alexander the Great's soldiers brought clay as a staple to ward off hunger and food poisoning; and in the Ukraine, bentonite clay and zeolites were used to decontaminate the surrounding area after the Chernobyl disaster.

Clay is an excellent "cleaner" that draws out toxins, such as chemicals, heavy metals, and free radicals, then binds with them through the electrical charges created between its layers. This pulls the toxins into the clay, eliminating them from the body. Clay face masks draw impurities from deep within the skin to leave it fresh, radiant, and glowing, with the added bonus of increasing collagen synthesis.

Here are some of clay's additional beauty benefits:

- Cleans and shrinks pores
- Hydrates and moisturizes skin
- Improves skin tone and elasticity
- Rejuvenates and regenerates the skin
- Exfoliates the skin
- Soothes sensitive skin
- Helps with diaper rash and redness

There are many different types of clay, including bentonite, rhassoul, French green, fuller's earth, and kaolin. Let's go through what the differences are and how to use them.

Bentonite clay is probably the most well-known of all the clays. It is formed after volcanic ash has weathered and aged in the presence of water and has a strong negative electromagnetic charge because it's missing an ion; therefore it seeks out toxins to bind with and complete itself. When activated by water, it functions like a magnet, drawing heavy metals and toxins to itself, neutralizing these volatile precursors to disease. An energy enhancer, it can aid in the oxygenation of cells by pulling excess hydrogen out of the cells; this can help to repair muscles after a hard workout. Bentonite is safe to take internally to remove heavy metal toxins and unwanted bacteria and viruses. Topically it's used to combat eczema, dermatitis, and psoriasis, and it's highly effective when mixed into a toothpaste or used as an ingredient in deodorant.

Bentonite Clay Detoxifying Mask

1 teaspoon bentonite clay

½ teaspoon dried herb of your choice, such as chamomile flowers (optional)

1 teaspoon raw organic honey

1 teaspoon spring water (the less water you use, the thicker the mask; add more as desired)

2 drops essential oil of your choice, such as lavender (optional)

In a small bowl, thoroughly combine the bentonite clay with the dried herb. Add the honey and form a thick paste. Add the water as needed to create a consistency that isn't too thick or thin (depending on your personal preference). Then add the essential oil.

Apply the mask immediately to your face and neck, avoiding your eyes. Leave it on until it has hardened, approximately 10 to 20 minutes.

Gently wash off the mask with a warm washcloth (the warmer the better since the heat helps take the mask off without you having to rub the skin). Pat your skin dry and then apply your favorite natural toner and moisturizer.

Rhassoul clay is a prized beauty ingredient that hails from the Atlas Mountains in Morocco, where it is formed through a combination of volcanic and geothermal activity. It has the unique ability to deeply clean the skin while nourishing it, so it can be used every day as a natural soap and shampoo. It is touted to even out skin tone and increase elasticity while reducing blemishes, dryness, redness, and flakiness. It is a great exfoliant when mixed with substances like salt, sugar, or oatmeal.

Often the choice of leading spas for hair and skin packs, rhassoul clay contains higher levels of minerals than most clays, like iron, lithium, magnesium, potassium, silica, sodium, and trace elements. Although it carries a similar negative electromagnetic charge as bentonite, unlike bentonite clay, rhassoul clay is best used topically and should only be used internally under the guidance of a medical professional.

French green clay, also known as "sea clay" or "illite," is a pretty clay that was used in ancient Egypt, Greece, and Rome to treat skin and support digestion. Able to be taken internally or used externally, sea clay is naturally high in several important mineral oxides, calcite, copper, dolomite, iron, magnesium, manganese, phosphorous, potassium, quartz, selenium, and silica. It is highly absorbent and excellent for tightening the pores due to its micromolecules, which drink up oils and impurities from the skin. It is used for a whole host of topical reasons for the hair and skin, including to calm inflammation, to improve the complexion, to remove dead skin cells, to stimulate blood flow to the skin, to reduce the appearance of facial scars, to minimize dark spots, to repair split ends, and to clean the scalp.

Fuller's earth clay, also known as "multani mitti," is most well-known for two reasons: its ability to absorb massive amounts of oil and its prowess at lightening the skin. This clay is so powerful at soaking up oil, it's now relied on by manufacturers to soak up spilled automobile oil and it's used as a main ingredient in kitty litter. Its powers of absorption can be put to work for you, drawing oils and impurities out of your skin when used in a face mask. It's an extremely strong material, so when used on the face, it's often mixed with some bentonite clay. Do not ingest this clay.

Kaolin clay, being the mildest of all clays, is suitable for people with sensitive skin. By stimulating circulation to the skin, it does not draw out oil but rather gently exfoliates and cleanses the skin. It contains a high amount of silica, which helps to remove dead skin cells, leading to regeneration and rejuvenation. In addition, kaolin clay has unique minerals and phytonutrients that create a nice moisture balance. It too should not be taken internally.

CHARCOAL

I have spent the past several years researching and experimenting with charcoal, and I firmly believe it is by far the simplest and most effective health and beauty element in history. Although charcoal is nothing new, I am inspired to share with you some of the astonishing facts and compelling science I have learned about this powerful substance.

Of all the detoxification strategies I have researched and used over the decades, both charcoal and clay are the simplest and easiest to implement in daily life with massive results. Since ancient times, both animals and humans have relied on charcoal to counteract the harmful effects of toxic materials that have been ingested, intentionally or otherwise.

How does charcoal work? Charcoal detoxifies because, like clay, it is negatively charged and absorptive like a sponge. Absorption is the adhesion of atoms, ions, or molecules from a gas, liquid, or dissolved solid to a surface. Toxic ions, materials, or molecules are typically positively charged, and the surface of the charcoal is negatively charged; therefore they are attracted to each other, and the toxic substance is consumed by the absorptive charcoal. If we don't pre-filter toxins and chemicals with charcoal, then in the next step we become the filter. I always say to people at my lectures, "Either get a filter or become a filter."

Charcoal is a lifesaving and longevity-inducing substance. Centuries' worth of evidence hints at the many beneficial qualities of charcoal. It is natural, safe, nontoxic, and may immediately relieve several ailments, including drug overdose, food poisoning, stomach flu, gas (flatulence), and stomach pain. A charcoal drink is the go-to treatment in emergency rooms after a suspected overdose or poisoning. One interesting study carried out even suggests charcoal may increase the life span of mammals by 43 percent.

Being porous and essentially chemically inert, charcoal solely depends upon its physical and electrochemical ability to trap toxins. It can bind to other compounds, including nearly every toxin (whether mineral or organic), odorous gases, and even microorganisms along with their waste. When ingested, charcoal pieces form toxin-charcoal complexes. Since the body cannot absorb or break down most charcoal pieces, because they are too large, the pieces are excreted through bowel movements along with the toxins they carry. The porous nature of the charcoal structure increases the surface area available for absorption, thereby enhancing the rate and capacity of detoxification: a piece of charcoal can absorb up to two hundred times its own weight in toxic material! Plus, since the foreign particles are safely trapped within the pores of the charcoal structure, digestive enzymes are prevented from reacting upon the toxins, thus eliminating the risk of poisons being remetabolized and reintroduced.

How do you use charcoal to remove toxins? You may not think to reach for activated charcoal when it's time to brush your teeth, but this powerful agent is actually one of the best oral cleaners out there. Smearing black powder on your teeth may seem counterintuitive, but the mighty cleansing action of activated charcoal in the mouth can't be denied for both toxin elimination and whitening prowess.

Just as charcoal helps to remove pathogens from our internal terrain, it does so for our mouth. When we rub activated charcoal around our teeth and gums, it acts like a highly absorbent sponge collecting toxins, surface stains, and bacteria to itself. It positively affects the pH in our mouth to aid in the fight against tooth decay, gingivitis, and bad breath. The many Americans who religiously use chemical-based tooth gels and strips to whiten their teeth can feel even better about the switch to charcoal. Without stripping off layers of enamel, charcoal truly cleans the teeth to reveal their natural shine. The warnings on regular toothpastes that say "harmful if swallowed" do not apply here either—if you swallow activated charcoal, it will just pass through your digestive system trapping more toxins as it goes before being eliminated!

Activated charcoal may be consumed as a supplement or applied with some water topically (such as to an insect bite). Activated char-

coal used to filter water acts to absorb chemicals, toxins, and pollutants. However, it is not self-cleaning; once its surface area is full of
compounds, it must be replaced.

I recommend starting off ingesting between 500 and 1,500 milligrams four or five times a week. If you have a sensitive digestive
tract, switch to just charcoal (not activated), which is less aggressive.
Once you are familiar with the regular use of charcoal and understand its effects on your digestion and body, you may want to occasionally increase to 5,000 to 10,000 milligrams when you require that
much.

Clean Sweep Charcoal Lemonade

2 cups coconut water or aloe vera juice
1 tablespoon chia seeds
¼ cup freshly squeezed lemon juice (about 2 medium lemons)
Stevia or raw organic honey to taste
2 capsules charcoal powder

*In a glass mason jar, combine 1 cup of the coconut water or aloe vera
juice and the chia seeds, shake the jar, and let the mixture sit for the
chia seeds to gel. After about 10 minutes, shake the jar again and add
the remaining cup of liquid as well as the lemon juice and sweetener.
Open the charcoal capsules and empty the contents into the jar, and
shake the jar again. Adjust for desired sweetness.*

Ingesting activated charcoal can sometimes cause constipation,
so adding demulcents like aloe vera and chia seeds, as in the Clean
Sweep Charcoal Lemonade recipe included here, helps keep things
moving. In addition, lemon juice is stimulating for peristalsis, and if

you use raw organic honey as a sweetener, it contains extra enzymes and minerals. Coconut water as a base is very hydrating, and aloe vera juice is soothing for the digestive system.

Note that consuming charcoal may turn your stools dark. It's best to consume this lemonade two hours before or after meals or taking other supplements. Charcoal may reduce the effects of medications too—and it may neutralize them completely. If you are taking medications or a hormone-based contraceptive, avoid ingesting charcoal within four to five hours of taking them.

Here are two other charcoal recipes for you to try:

Vanilla Charcoal Latte

This is a great bedtime drink—best enjoyed two hours before or after eating or taking other supplements.

12 ounces organic coconut milk

2 to 3 teaspoons raw organic honey

½ teaspoon vanilla powder

2 capsules charcoal powder

Pinch of Celtic or Icelandic sea salt

In a saucepan, gently warm the coconut milk until it starts to bubble but not boil.

In a high-speed blender, combine the warmed coconut milk with the honey, vanilla powder, charcoal powder, and salt, and blend the mixture until it's creamy.

Note: You can open and empty the charcoal capsule powder into the blender or simply drop the whole charcoal capsules into the warmed coconut milk and the capsules will dissolve.

Activated Charcoal Mask

Only three ingredients!

1 teaspoon bentonite clay

1 teaspoon activated charcoal

1 to 2 teaspoons apple cider vinegar (depending on the desired consistency of the mask)

Combine all the ingredients in a bowl, and with clean fingers, spread the paste all over your clean, dry face and neck in a circular motion, avoiding your eyes. Let it sit for 15 minutes.

Rinse your face with cool water and then apply your favorite toner and moisturizer.

INFRARED

Infrared is a light spectrum consisting of a group of invisible heating waves that can be absorbed directly by your body's molecules without significantly increasing the temperature of the air around you—such as what you would experience in an infrared sauna.

Perhaps the most exciting scientific breakthrough in infrared therapy came from a study in which researchers employed a combination of infrared light, bipolar radiofrequency, and vacuum and mechanical massage. Twenty-nine subjects, between the ages of twenty-eight and seventy, received four weeks of treatments on either their upper arms or their abdomens and the sides of their torsos (flanks). This study showed, with statistical significance, that this treatment modality acts upon cellulite to produce a lasting reduction in circumference and improvement in appearance without surgical or pharmaceutical intervention.

How does infrared work on fat? Fat-soluble toxins bind to fat cells and are stored in clusters of fatty tissue. In order for the body to rid itself of these sticky toxins, it has to filter them through the liver and transform them into water-soluble metabolites. These metabolites will then typically follow a pathway out of the body through bile (bowels), sweat, or urine. The first step toward mobilizing them is breaking them free from the fat clusters they form (cellulite), and the study proved that infrared treatments can play an important role in that.

For anyone who is overweight or obese, it is essential to understand that the fat cells in your body may harbor harmful, undesirable toxins that can cause disease. When you take the steps I've recommended in *The Beauty Diet*, you're likely to begin seeing fat loss, and whenever you lose fat, you're potentially releasing fat-soluble toxins back into your bloodstream unmetabolized. You must work with your body and your liver to turn these fat-solubles into water-soluble metabolites. This will enable your body to excrete the toxins.

I believe treatments using the infrared spectrum, particularly far infrared, are key in this type of detoxification. Not only does infrared accelerate detoxification, it greatly improves circulation and blood flow to the skin, delivering vital nutrients that help it shine. Many holistic health practitioners offer long-duration infrared sauna sessions at reasonable prices. I recommend easing into the practice when you're first starting out. Begin with ten- to twenty-minute sessions for several days at 110 degrees Fahrenheit, then slowly add to the duration and temperature until you can comfortably remain in the sauna for an hour at 130 degrees Fahrenheit.

CONCLUSION

We are exposed to an unprecedented amount of human-made toxins in today's world. The body has not yet adapted to being able to remove all of them—we must help it. From one point of view, detoxification is more important than nutrition. Detoxification is critical for beauty. By supporting and optimizing the body's natural cleansing pathways, you can experience better health, weight management, high levels of energy, and elevated mood so you can look and feel your best in this chemically challenged world. As the body slowly ages, it accumulates more and more toxins. Engaging in regular, consistent detoxification over your lifetime in a relaxed and balanced manner will ensure that your body never becomes overwhelmed or overburdened.

Please see the detoxifying Three-Day Beauty Cleanse later in the book (page 235) to reboot your body's systems and enable that healthy, youthful glow!

Detox, not Botox. That's a motto to live by.

Nourish Cells

Beauty begins with our cells.

Our cells come in all different shapes and sizes, and are the basic building blocks by which organs, tissues, and blood are created. The body is composed of 30 trillion cells, which constantly communicate with one another to help the body respond to its environment based on what we touch, smell, and eat. They protect our DNA while providing structure for the body, and they undertake the important job of turning nutrients from food into energy, which fuels the cellular processes to develop our physical appearance.

Within the center of each cell are many tightly coiled bundles of DNA called chromosomes. Each chromosome contains thousands of genes, which came from our parents. These genes call out detailed instructions to create all different kinds of proteins used by the cell to form everything that makes me look like me, and you look like you. How much collagen we have in our skin, how thick our hair is, how strong our nails are—chromosomes determine all this and more.

Cells need to be nourished and hydrated properly in order to function well. When we lack a proper balance of sleep, exercise, and minerals and vitamins, our cells cannot operate efficiently, and it is reflected in our appearance. The function of tissues and organs becomes compromised, and we see this clearly with split nails, brittle hair, dry skin, acne, dull eyes, discolored teeth, foot fungus, eczema . . . the list goes on. These are all indications that our cells are missing the proper cellular food for our organs and tissues to thrive.

To radiate beauty from the inside out, we need flawless cellular function, and that is determined by four things:

- Cellular nutrition
- Cellular protection
- Cellular hydration
- Cellular optimization

CELLULAR NUTRITION

In order to grow and function properly, cells require a host of nutrients. We need to ensure that we get an adequate amount of vitamins and minerals each day in order to maintain the integrity of our cells to support strong teeth, hair, nails, and skin. We *can* feed our cells to function at their maximum capacity both healthwise and beautywise, so let's dig into what nutrients support beauty and what foods support health on a cellular level.

VITAMINS

Vitamins are potent nutrients that can prevent and even reverse the aging of the skin, boost hydration, increase collagen production, brighten the eyes, and strengthen the hair, teeth, and nails. They

can be obtained through organic whole foods and are critical to both
beauty and health.

There are two classes of vitamins: fat-soluble and water-soluble.
The water-soluble vitamins are the B-complex vitamins and vitamin C.
Fat-soluble vitamins include A, D, E, and K and require the presence
of lipids to be absorbed. Let's take a look at some of these powerhouse
beauty building blocks.

Vitamin A (beta-carotene) is a beauty enhancer both systemically and
topically. When used directly on the skin, it has antibacterial properties, which aid in the healing of acne and rosacea. It also improves
the appearance of the skin, promoting healing from photodamage and
reversing hyperpigmentation.

When ingested, vitamin A nourishes the skin and the hair. It also
reverses UV damage and may even prevent it when taken before exposure to damaging light. In the human body and in an animal's body,
beta-carotene and certain other carotenoids transform into vitamin
A (retinoids) including retinol, retinal, and retinoic acids. These play
a key role in immune function. Retinoic acid deeply hydrates the hair
and scalp.

Raw organic carrots, green leafy vegetables (kale, chard, etc.),
pumpkins, squash, and sweet potatoes provide a healthy dose of the
beauty-enhancing benefits of the precursor to vitamin A (retinoids):
beta-carotene. Animal products such as eggs and ghee already contain vitamin A forms (retinoids) that do not need to be transformed by
your digestion and are immediately available as nutrition to your cells.

Vitamin B_9 (folate or folic acid) is essential for the formation and
repair of DNA, especially promoting healthy replication and repair of
skin cells that have been harmed by UV rays. When combined with
vitamin B_{12} and UVB sun exposure, folic acid stimulates the precur-

sors to melanocytes, which can then travel to the epidermis and reverse vitiligo (loss of pigment in the skin).

Topically, vitamin B_9 is best used in conjunction with creatine to increase collagen gene expression, collagen production, and collagen fibril organization, all of which promote the reduction of wrinkles and fine lines.

The best foods to eat for vitamin B_9 are raw organic beets, broccoli, celery, lentils, strawberries, sweet bell peppers, and tomatoes.

Vitamin B_{12}, a water-soluble vitamin, is a DNA protector when combined with vitamin B_9 (folate or folic acid). Together, these two prevent chromosome breakage and DNA hypomethylation, a key abnormality in human cancer tumors. On its own, vitamin B_{12} promotes blood circulation, delivering oxygen and nutrients to the surface of the skin, resulting in the reversal of epidermis damage and the emergence of smooth, fresh skin. It contributes to bone, brain, and nervous system health, and also keeps our energy levels up.

Plants don't have the ability to process and store B_{12} within themselves like animals do, so it's important to consider taking a B_{12} supplement when eating a primarily plant-based diet. Vitamin B_{12} is found in eggs, cheese, poultry, fish, and meat. Vegans must rely upon supplementation to maintain healthy levels.

Vitamin C packs a beauty punch, promoting healthy, glowing skin by boosting collagen production and optimizing the immune system. Studies have shown that vitamin C congregates at both the epidermal and the dermal layers of the skin and has been shown to repair UV-related DNA damage, prevent oxidative damage to lipids, inhibit the release of inflammatory cytokines, and protect against cell death. In these ways, as levels of vitamin C drop in the skin, signs of wear and tear begin to emerge.

Vitamin C is found in an abundance of beauty foods, including raw organic amla berries, citrus fruits, guava, kiwi, papaya, pineapple, red pepper, seabuckthorn berries, strawberries, and more. Because this water-soluble vitamin is not made by our body nor stored easily and is quickly excreted, it is important to consume these foods regularly.

Vitamin D is essential for absorbing many other beauty nutrients. Vitamin D, specifically Vitamin D_3, is perhaps the most important vitamin for human health, as it flips on over three thousand genes associated with health. Because it regulates calcium and phosphorus absorption it plays a pivotal role in bone health, and deficiencies can lead to osteoporosis. This fat-soluble vitamin functions like a hormone and interacts with our DNA. It also repairs and strengthens skin, rendering it resistant to sun damage.

Because vitamin D reduces inflammation and supports the immune system it is considered an "anti-acne" vitamin. Vitamin D is so important that it is used to fortify everything from milk to orange juice. Despite this fortification, almost a third of the American population is deficient in vitamin D. Staying indoors and leading a sedentary lifestyle will reduce your sun exposure and vitamin D_3 production, leading to reduced energy, a weaker immune system, and sallow looking skin.

Vitamin D_3 is produced through sun exposure and supports a healthy immune system, weight loss, and even mood. Top tips for getting enough vitamin D_3 include getting twenty minutes of direct sun exposure a day (don't shower for at least thirty minutes after exposure to allow absorption into the skin). Foods like salmon and sardines can be used as food sources of vitamin D, and although vegetarian sources are hard to come by (small amounts of vitamin D_2 are present in lichens; shiitake, maitake, and portobello mushrooms; as well as polypores like reishi and chaga that are dried in the sun), there are vegan vitamin D_2 and lichen-derived vitamin D_3 supplements available—and vitamin D_2 may be as powerful as vitamin D_3.

Vitamin E, when taken internally, has potent anti-inflammatory properties and acts like an antioxidant to prevent free-radical damage within our cells. This boosts moisture and elasticity, resulting in youthful-looking skin due to faster cellular regeneration. While working hard against wrinkles, scars, and acne, it also helps block environmental damage to the hair. There are eight different types of vitamin E (all with their unique benefits): four types of tocopherols and four types of tocotrienols (derived from rice bran solubles)— and all are beneficial and recommended for beauty. Topically, the alpha-tocopherols are isolated from vitamin E and infused into beauty creams and oils for their humectant properties. They excel at hydrating and smoothing dry nail beds and cuticles, lubricating the skin, and adding shine to the hair. Vitamin E is abundant in healthy fats and can be found in almonds, avocados (of course), hemp seeds, organic cold-pressed extra-virgin olive oil, and sunflower seeds, as well as in asparagus, beet greens, kale, mustard greens, spinach, and swiss chard.

Vitamin K is another fat-soluble vitamin that is a beauty enhancer. It is essential for the promotion of platelet aggregation (blood clotting), and it improves blood circulation, helping the body heal from wounds and bruises, including dark circles under the eyes. Vitamin K has also been shown to prevent calcification of the elastin fibers in the skin. This in turn prevents the formation of wrinkles. It can also prevent further acne outbreaks. Eat raw organic brussels sprouts, cabbage, celery, kale, scallions, and spinach to get plenty of vitamin K.

Vitamin K_2 assists with calcium regulation and can affect our dental health. Vitamin K_2 protects the heart and cardiovascular system from soft tissue calcification. Because K_2 is found primarily in dairy cheese, fermented soybean products (e.g., natto), fermented nut and seed products, as well as supplements, all of us need to pay particular attention to K_2 levels, especially in developing children. Vitamin K_2 and vitamin D work together to produce strong bone health.

SuperVitaSmoothie

This smoothie is a very satisfying breakfast or meal replacement because it provides so much dense nutritional sustenance in a delicious fruity beverage.

12 ounces coconut milk

1 whole orange, peeled and seeded

1 cup fresh or frozen raspberries

Small handful of baby spinach or kale

2 tablespoons tocotrienols

1 tablespoon chia seeds

Contents of 1 to 2 capsules vitamin C

¼ teaspoon vanilla powder

1 to 2 dates, pitted; raw organic honey; or stevia to taste

Blend all the ingredients together in a high-speed blender and enjoy!

MINERALS

Beauty depends on mineralization: minerals govern 95 percent of the body's activities! Major and trace minerals allow the nearly four thousand enzymes (small proteins) contained in each cell to fully function, fueling every cell to work to its fullest potential. Without hardworking enzymes, the body is unable to completely break down nutrients for absorption and waste products for elimination, which leads to weight gain, inflammation, digestive distress, fatigue—and all of this affects how we look to the rest of the world.

Many people have not activated each of these four thousand enzymes in their body because they do not have enough minerals in their diet. If minerals come through in the form of plants, then the body can assimilate them and utilize them immediately. The following are some of the most important minerals required by the body to create and maintain beauty:

Iron deficiency leads to a decrease in red blood cell production. Reduction of red blood cells leads to a decrease in oxygen and nutrients delivered to the skin cells. A decrease in oxygen and nutrients leads to pale, wan, sickly skin. Low iron stores can also result in limp, dull hair and hair loss.

On the flip side, a diet rich in iron ensures delivery of all the nutrients and oxygen necessary for cultivating beauty at a cellular level as well as right on the surface of the skin. Iron speeds wound healing, nourishes tissues, and improves hair texture.

The best sources of natural plant-based iron include organic beans (e.g., black beans, lentils), cacao (e.g., dark chocolate), green vegetables (e.g., broccoli, chard, dandelion, kale, spinach), seeds (e.g., pumpkin seeds, squash seeds), the skins of many different fruits and vegetables (e.g., sweet potato), and sunflower family roots (e.g., Jerusalem artichokes, yacon root). Animal foods are typically rich in iron; red meat, for example, is red due to the iron-rich blood of the animal.

Magnesium has many beauty benefits, some direct and some indirect. Indirectly, magnesium promotes sleep, calm, and stress reduction by opening up hundreds of detoxification pathways. It also reduces swelling, eases joint pain, and relieves muscle spasms and pain. This keeps you moving and grooving in harmony and peace with yourself and with the earth. Directly, magnesium detoxifies and cleanses the skin, calming allergic skin reactions, reducing fine lines and wrinkles, strengthening hair follicles and hair strands, and preventing hair loss. When applied topically, magnesium is easily absorbed through the skin. While at first it may cause an uncomfortable itching (a sign of systemic deficiency), in the long run it reduces swelling, heals cracked heels, prevents odor in the armpits, combats acne, and stimulates the lymphatic system, which enhances the growth of new skin cells.

Magnesium is most abundantly found in avocado, dark leafy greens (e.g., chard, kale, spinach), magnesium sulfate, nuts (e.g., almonds, cashews, pistachios), pumpkin seeds, sea salt, and of course my favorite—chocolate.

Selenium can be applied topically or taken internally. Topically, it works as an antioxidant and anti-inflammatory, soothing redness and sensitivity as well as acting as a natural skin toner. It also combats yeasts and fungi, particularly those that cause dandruff and itchy discoloration of the scalp.

Taken internally, selenium reduces skin inflammation and UV cell damage, protects against hyperpigmentation, and inhibits inflammatory cytokines that break down collagen in the skin. It also mobilizes white blood cells, enhancing their response to infections on and beneath the skin.

Selenium is found naturally in beans (e.g., lima, pinto), Brazil nuts (variable, but still the best source), brown or black rice, mushrooms (e.g., button, cremini, shiitake), seeds (e.g., chia, sesame, sunflower), and vegetables (e.g., broccoli, cabbage, spinach). Some of the most toxin-contaminated seafoods (e.g., clams, lobster, mussels) and fish (e.g., tilapia, tuna) are rich in selenium but simply no longer trustworthy as food sources.

Sulfur is foundational to beauty. Adequate sulfur intake ensures a beautiful complexion, mineralized hair, and glowing skin. High concentrations of sulfur promote cell division, cell repair, cell growth, and the production of T-lymphocyte white blood cells. Sulfur is also vital for the formation of fat-digesting bile and the regulation of blood sugar.

Sulfur's most essential beauty contribution, though, is in the formation of collagen, which retains fluid and provides elasticity and flexibility to all the tissues of the body, including the skin. Sulfur compounds, like glucosamine, give connective tissue its strength, ensuring strong bones, ligaments, tendons, skin, eyes, and nails. Sulfur is also found in keratin, the fibrous protein that protects hair and nails from damage and stress.

MSM (methylsulfonylmethane) is an organic sulfur compound typically found as a crystalized powder (but also found in a non-oxidized liquid form, for topical use, known as DMSO) that makes sulfur bioavailable to nearly every type of tissue. One of its primary beauty functions is to produce the powerful antioxidant glutathione, which binds to heavy metals and other toxins and carries them out of the body. MSM also breaks up bad calcium, preventing arthritis, repairing scar tissue that is too rich in hardened nitrogen, and repairing damaged cartilage. Furthermore, MSM promotes insulin production, encouraging healthy blood sugar levels. Experts have dubbed MSM the "beauty supplement" for good reason since it supports collagen and keratin production, both essential for healthy skin, nails, and hair.

When applied topically and mixed in lotions, MSM and other sulfur compounds prevent acne, seborrheic dermatitis, rosacea, dandruff, and eczema. Sulfur lotions are powerful exfoliants and can be used to effectively treat tissue damaged by warts, skin discoloration, shingles, psoriasis, split heels, and hair follicle infections. The best sources of sulfur include bok choy, broccoli, cabbage, cauliflower, chives, eggs, garlic, hemp seeds, kale, MSM, nuts, onions, seeds, spirulina, and more. You can increase your chances of obtaining healthy levels of sulfur naturally by eating wild plants and mushrooms, as these are dependent on natural rainfall, which replenishes the soil with minerals such as sulfur.

Zinc may come last alphabetically, but when it comes to beauty, it deserves position number one. It is crucial for detoxification, nourishing the lymphatic organs and promoting premium liver function. Through this process, it aids with tissue repair and oxygenation. When taken with vitamin A and sulfur, it builds strong, lustrous hair. When taken with vitamin E, it supports healthy reproductive systems in both men and women, raising sexual energy and generating more sex appeal.

Along with nearly every other vitamin and mineral mentioned here, zinc is part of the recipe for stimulating collagen production. It is also essential to the enzymes that digest damaged collagen, making way for the repair of collagen. In so doing, zinc prevents wrinkles, stretch marks, and the outward signs of skin distress.

Zinc also works topically for the treatment of acne and the reduction of skin inflammation from rashes, allergies, and other types of contact dermatitis. It is perhaps the only topical sunscreen option that provides broad-spectrum sun protection with the added benefits of supporting beauty rather than detracting from it the way chemical sunscreens do. It locks in moisture, prevents bacterial infections and acne, and reduces dandruff and inflammatory skin ailments, like rosacea. It also supports recovery from burns and the repair of damaged tissues.

Add zinc to your diet by eating an abundance of beans (e.g., chickpeas/hummus, kidney), black foods (e.g., black beans, black rice, black tahini), mushrooms, nuts (e.g., raw organic cacao, cashews), seeds (e.g., pumpkin seeds, watermelon seeds), and vegetables (e.g., spinach, garlic).

CELLULAR PROTECTION

Damage to our cells influences visual aging. Important compounds in the body mitigate cellular damage, and when we fuel ourselves with healthy foods and make lifestyle choices to support those compounds, we can maintain our cells as long as possible. The older the body gets, the less it is able to protect itself on its own from the damaging effects of free radicals and inflammation, so it becomes more important to support the body's cells in the most helpful and positive ways.

ANTIOXIDANTS

Free radicals are highly reactive compounds that bind to cells, harming and destroying them. The body naturally creates free radicals (oxidative stress) through the process of metabolism and when it needs to kill off viruses and bacteria. Free radicals cause skin to have brown spots and become saggy, and they break down the skin's collagen, which causes wrinkles. The great news is the body naturally creates antioxidants too, which mitigate the damage of oxidative stress by cleaning up the free radicals before they can do serious harm. Antioxidants prevent cell damage, rapid aging, and inflammation.

Unfortunately, we also take in free radicals when we breathe in pollution or cigarette smoke, or come into contact with herbicides or radiation, so the body easily becomes overrun with them. We need to actively take in more antioxidants from food, herbs, and water, and through the nutrients we put on our skin directly, to balance out the overabundance of free radicals.

A visual example of free-radical damage and oxidative stress is when an avocado turns brown. When you squeeze a lemon on it (which contains vitamin C), the avocado stops browning. This is because the lemon contains antioxidants.

Total Cell Antioxidant Blast

12 to 16 ounces coconut nettle tea (see instructions)

1 3.5-ounce packet frozen acai

½ cup fresh or frozen blueberries

½ cup fresh or frozen strawberries

Small handful of fresh spinach

1 tablespoon hemp seeds

1 tablespoon chia seeds

1 tablespoon goji berries

1 tablespoon cacao powder

1 to 2 teaspoons maca powder

Raw organic honey to taste

Use coconut water as the base to make the nettle tea. (Or substitute spring water if preferred, but coconut water is very hydrating.) Allow the tea to cool, then refrigerate it until you're ready to use it.

Blend the chilled coconut nettle tea with all the remaining ingredients in a high-speed blender, and enjoy the mixture cold.

FREE RADICALS AND OXIDATIVE STRESS

Free radicals are molecules with unpaired electrons, which makes them unstable. They can damage other cells and tissues around them by trying to steal an extra electron from the atoms. Antioxidants donate an electron to a free radical so the free radical doesn't have to steal an electron from other cells.

In order to maintain a youthful appearance, free-radical damage should be reduced as much as possible. Many people devote lots of time to intense exercise in an effort to look thin and beautiful. However, in order to exercise, the body's cells need to produce energy, and when mitochondria produce energy (adenosine triphosphate, or ATP), the side effect is oxidative stress. If someone with a high-carb diet full of white bread, pasta, and other high-glycemic foods hits the gym for a high-intensity workout to counter the effects, that person actually fuels a vicious cycle of rapid aging and free-radical damage to his or her body instead of accomplishing the goal of youth and beauty.

To make sure you keep your antioxidants high enough to handle the number of free radicals in your body, try to incorporate these natural, high-ORAC-score foods into your diet as often as possible. An "oxygen radical absorbance capacity" rating is determined by a lab test that quantifies the food's total antioxidant capacity—basically how much it will protect your cells against the free radicals in your body. The higher the score, the more protective it is.

- Goji berries: 25,000 ORAC score*
- Cacao (chocolate): 21,000 ORAC score
- Pecans: 17,000 ORAC score
- Wild blueberries: 14,000 ORAC score
- Elderberries: 14,000 ORAC score
- Cranberries: 9,500 ORAC score
- Artichokes: 9,400 ORAC score
- Kidney beans: 8,400 ORAC score
- Blackberries: 5,300 ORAC score
- Cilantro: 5,100 ORAC score

The top three antioxidants I recommend in addition to the foods in the previous list are resveratrol, astaxanthin, and glutathione.

---

* Scores approximated from the Nutrient Data Laboratory, Beltsville Human Nutrition Research Center, part of the Agricultural Research Service of the US Department of Agriculture.

Resveratrol is a yellow flavonoid and super nutrient found in the skin of grapes, some red wines, peanuts, and some berries. It is a polyphenol that acts as an antioxidant to blast inflammation and reduce bad cholesterol. It is believed to activate the anti-aging gene Sirtuin 1 (*SIRT1*) and is touted as the primary molecule behind the "French paradox," which infers that French citizens live about twenty years longer than average among industrialized countries due to their intake of dark red wine.

Astaxanthin is a red carotenoid pigment found in certain marine plants (plankton and algae) and animals (krill, salmon, red trout, shrimp, crab, and lobster) as well as dark leafy greens. Often called the "king of the carotenoids," astaxanthin is recognized as one of the most powerful antioxidants in nature. It is especially protective against oxidation and is a hefty free-radical scavenger, providing additional benefits for eye health, nervous system strength, and joint lubrication.

Glutathione (GSH) is a peptide made up of three amino acids that every cell in the body produces, which makes it our most important

---

Mitochondria

Mitochondria are the powerhouses in cells. They take in fat, sugar, and protein from food, combine them with oxygen, and turn them into usable energy for the cells and tissues. They contain their own genetic material, separate from the nucleus, which is critical to the energy creation process, and can make copies of themselves if the body needs more energy created. When the body has too many free radicals, mitochondria can become damaged over time, leading to chronic fatigue.

antioxidant. Scientists believe that it is so critical to overall health that the length of a person's life can be predicted by the level of GSH in that person's cells. GSH deficiency causes cells to be more vulnerable to oxidative stress and chronic disease, while higher levels of GSH help T-cell function and cell detoxification in the immune system. Glutathione-creating substances can be found in milk thistle; avocado; sulfur-rich veggies (broccoli, cauliflower, kale, etc.); vitamins B_6, B_9, B_{12}, C, and E; biotin; and selenium.

ESSENTIAL FATTY ACIDS

During digestion, the body breaks down the fats you eat into fatty acids, which are then used to fuel the cells for all their daily activities when glucose isn't available. Cells also have the important job of creating phospholipids, which are an essential component of all cell membranes and precursors to prostaglandins, which regulate inflammation.

There are a number of essential fatty acids—the building blocks for beautiful, glowing, radiant skin. The body must acquire EFAs from your diet, including linoleic acid as well as alpha-linolenic acid,

Cell Membrane

Surrounding each cell is a protective cell membrane, a plasma membrane. This is mainly composed of fats (with some proteins) and functions like a drop of oil in the heavily water-based bloodstream to keep each cell segregated from its environment. The membrane acts like a filter, allowing nutrients to enter and wastes to exit, and the cell creates energy without interruption. The membrane is the walkie-talkie, so to speak, that enables each cell to communicate with one another, orchestrating physiological functions seamlessly. This is why eating healthy fats is *so* important in your diet!

eicosapentaenoic acid (EPA), and docosahexaenoic acid (DHA). You will know these by their more popular names: omega-3 and omega-6 fatty acids. Omega-3s, in particular, are like an inner moisturizer. They nourish hair follicles and create healthy, clear skin and strong, lustrous nails. They are also natural antioxidants and reduce oxidative damage and inflammation inside the cell, which occurs with daily metabolic function.

The important thing to understand about EFAs is that you need them in the proper ratio. Many of us get *plenty* of omega-6s but are deficient in omega-3s. The recommendation is to eat a one-to-one omega-6 to omega-3 ratio. Due to the high levels of vegetable oils used in processed foods, Americans can have an elevated ratio of up to twenty to one omega-6s to omega-3s, which promotes inflammation. This is catastrophic for health and beauty! Omega-6 fatty acids are present in almonds, Brazil nuts, canola oil, corn oil, palm oil, peanuts, pine nuts, pumpkin seeds, soybeans and soy oil, sunflower seeds and oil, walnuts, and wheat germ, plus poultry and eggs, so you can see why the American diet is so omega-6 heavy.

When the EFA balance is off, the human body suffers at a cellular level, affecting every aspect of health, beauty, and longevity. Deficiency in EFAs, or a disruption in the balance between the two types, can result in dry, scaly, flaky skin; cracked, peeling fingernails; dandruff; dull hair; eczema; hay fever; or hives. This imbalance can also lead to coronary heart disease, stroke, Crohn's disease, ADHD, and more.

My motto is Nix the Six, particularly when talking about the processed sources of omega-6. With fatty acids, a little bit goes a long way. A handful of omega-6 nuts or seeds every day, and you're good to go, *as long as* you balance it with omega-3s. Healthy vegan sources of omega-3s include brussels sprouts, chia seeds, chlorella, dark leafy greens, and hemp seeds and oil.

HOW TO COMBAT
INFLAMMATION IN THE BODY

Inflammation occurs on a cellular level and can either be your friend or your foe. When inflammation is your friend, it is acting on behalf of your immune system to maintain, defend, and protect you. The cells of your immune system mobilize to the site of injury and widen the local blood vessels, causing a rush of fluid and immune cells into the surrounding tissues. Once the injury has been taken care of, the inflammation goes away and your body returns to normal.

When inflammation is your foe it continues unchecked and wreaks havoc on your body, such as in the case of an autoimmune condition. It causes major damage to your cells, which in turn destroys your physical appearance with puffy eyes, dark circles, saggy skin, fine lines, wrinkles, acne, redness, swelling, bloating, pigmentation change in the skin, and worse. Inflammation is the cause of a whole host of serious health conditions, including heart disease, arthritis, kidney disease, IBS, liver disease, Alzheimer's, diabetes, eczema, allergies . . . the list, unfortunately, goes on and on. Inflammation is now believed to be the underlying cause of more than eighty chronic diseases. "Inflammation may turn out to be the elusive Holy Grail of medicine—the single phenomenon that holds the key to sickness and health," William Meggs, MD, PhD, of East Carolina University stated in his book *The Inflammation Cure* (2003). Inflammation is so damaging and has been linked so strongly with the diseases of aging that scientists have coined the term "inflamm-aging."

Diet, stress, hormones, environment, and telomere damage all contribute to inflammation in the body. Fortunately, there are two major things you can do to fight it:

1. Avoid Inflammatory Foods

The fatty high-carbohydrate foods found in the Standard American Diet inflame your gut and your cells, contributing to low energy, toxic buildup, and bloating. Glucose from refined carbohydrates (white bread, pasta, white rice, alcohol, etc.) launches into your bloodstream and catapults your blood glucose. This increases the inflammatory messengers in your blood, called cytokines, which causes your immune system cells to divide faster to mitigate the inflammation. This causes physical cellular damage over time, reducing the telomeres within your cells. As telomeres get shorter, they start sending out steady inflammatory panic signals, and a vicious cycle ensues—your immune system cells divide faster to mitigate the inflammation, causing more telomere damage, causing more inflammation. See the problem here?

The best way to alleviate this detrimental downward inflammatory spiral is to completely eliminate inflammatory foods from your diet. We discussed in detail which foods to avoid and which to include in your diet in the "Eat for Beauty" chapter, but the top inflammatory foods to avoid are alcohol, artificial food additives, fast foods, fried foods, conventional grain-fed meat, dairy, MSG, refined cooking oils, refined flour, soda, and sugar.

Eating whole, organic, unprocessed foods will fight inflammation and inflamm-aging. Here are some examples of food groups to consider including in your diet: fermented/cultured foods, fruits (especially berries), green vegetables, nuts and seeds (eat more seeds than nuts and eat moderately), root vegetables, seaweeds, sprouts, superfoods, and superherbs.

2. Grounding/Earthing

> *In all things of Nature there is something of the marvelous.*
>
> —Aristotle

There is no inflammation in nature. This insight has profound implications for beauty and health when we understand the reason why.

The surface of the earth is *negatively* charged. In fact, it has trillions of negatively charged electrons teeming on the surface at all times. Inflammation can only occur in a body that is *positively* charged. When a body doesn't consistently touch the earth, it swings into a positive state, and this is the point at which inflammation takes hold.

As an "advanced" society, we have cleverly invented synthetic-soled shoes to protect our feet, but they also insulate us from the earth. We live in houses and buildings that keep us warm and dry, but they separate us further from the ground. We do group yoga in parks and place our plastic mats on the grass beneath us . . . even avid campers sleep on a thin layer of plastic, which stops the beneficial electrons of the earth from flowing into their bodies.

On top of that, we are bombarded by electromagnetic fields from our continuously advancing technologies. Computers, cell phones, TVs, and Wi-Fi keep us connected and entertained but are constantly throwing positively charged electricity at us throughout the day and night. Even our lamps and clocks are always projecting an electric field at us, including when turned off. When the body is directly connected to the earth, it is shielded from the electropollution of the present-day world. Never before has it been more critical to connect ourselves daily with the healing powers of the earth.

It's important to remember that the body is electrical before it is chemical. Electrical charges and impulses course through the body as the nervous system communicates with the brain to control all its basic biological functions. If the system is too positively charged, the body won't work properly, because the system will be overrun with free radicals and inflammation.

Touching the ground directly with the skin discharges any positive electricity built up during the day; at the same time, the body absorbs

---

Surfaces

Surfaces that will ground you: bare soil, ceramic tile, concrete (as long as it's not painted or sealed), copper, grass (preferably moist), leather, metal (like carbon or silver), sand.

Surfaces that will not ground you: anything synthetic (foam, glass, porcelain, etc.), asphalt, plastic, rubber, tar or tarmac, vinyl, wood.

---

millions of negatively charged electrons. These are like firefighters with a gigantic hose rushing in to douse the fires of inflammation, thickened blood, and heightened cortisol. This creates the perfect starting point for natural beauty to arise.

In today's world, it is quite easy to go days, weeks, even months without actually touching the earth. All the while, we scratch our heads, wondering why we are suffering from the growing inflammation adversely affecting how we look and feel.

Our ancestors aged gracefully without battling the chronic diseases we do today, and one of the major reasons was they were always outside. They walked barefoot on the earth or wore leather-soled shoes, a conductive material that gave them protection but still allowed the electrons to flow into their bodies. They also slept in direct contact with the earth or with only a conductive material between them.

I live part-time at my organic farm and research facility in Hawaii. I walk around and see locals in their sixties and seventies with slender builds, six-pack abs, lustrous hair, and youthful appearances. I used to assume it was from their surfing all day or engaging in physical labor. Over time, I came to realize it's the combination of a diet of unprocessed foods, exercise, and constant contact with the earth that gives them their extraordinary beauty and physique.

How often do you connect to the earth? When is the last time your bare feet touched the actual ground beneath you? Try to get at least twenty minutes of direct contact to the earth every single day, with forty minutes or more being optimal.

CHAGA: NATURE'S ANTI-INFLAMMATORY

I'm a mushroom hunter. Mushroom hunting season is absolutely my favorite season. There is nothing like being out in the woods consciously seeking out Mother Nature's best offerings to balance my state of health. Though technically a fungal mycelium, not a mushroom, chaga is something I avidly hunt for when I'm in Canada, because it grows in the cold-weather forests of the north where I spend my winters.

You won't find chaga on the ground; instead, you need to look high up in the trees, where, if you're lucky, you'll come across a big burned-looking, charcoal-like growth with a hard exterior that looks nothing like a mushroom.

Considered to be the "king of medicinal mushrooms," chaga was noted to be part of Chinese medicinal practice as early as the first century BCE. In Eastern Europe, chaga was traditionally used to treat skin conditions, like eczema. Many studies over the past few decades have demonstrated chaga's antibacterial, anti-inflammatory, anti-tumor, antioxidant, and hepatoprotective (liver-protective) properties, making it a powerful herb to have in your health and beauty repertoire.

Typically chaga grows on birch trees; it absorbs a beneficial compound from the birch called betulin, which has been shown to decrease inflammation and has antibacterial, antiseptic, and antiviral properties. Betulin is also heart protective and can help break down bad LDL cholesterol.

Chaga naturally contains ergosterol peroxide, which has been shown to be antitumor, anti-inflammatory, and antiviral. It contains beta glucans too, which further reduce inflammation and promote immune function.

Chaga also rates among the highest in antioxidants on the ORAC chart. Boiling a chunk of dried chaga with water produces a deep brown tea rich in melanin, an antioxidant that protects DNA from damage and is the main pigment in skin. Melanin works to keep skin supple and reduce wrinkles, and it can help protect skin from the damaging effects of UV rays.

Another antioxidant chaga offers is superoxide dismutase. Chaga's large quantities of SOD make it extremely helpful in neutralizing damage done by free radicals, which in turn slows the physical signs of the aging process. Chaga has up to fifty times more SOD than do leafy greens, fruits, and seaweeds.

In addition to all this, chaga is an adaptogen and helps the body combat stress, balancing all the body systems so hormones don't shift into overdrive, which taxes the adrenals and causes unnecessary damage and fatigue. Chaga is one superherb you're going to want to add to your daily beauty arsenal to roll back the effects of aging.

Superherb Chai

1 cup water

2 cups nut milk or coconut milk

2 teaspoons chai spice mix (cinnamon, cardamom, cloves, and ginger)

2 teaspoons maca powder

1 teaspoon chaga powder

Pinch of ground black pepper

Small pinch of sea salt

Raw organic honey

In a small saucepan combine the water and your choice of milk, and bring the mixture to a boil. Stir in the chai spice, maca, chaga, and black pepper. Cover the saucepan and simmer the chai for 20 minutes.

Strain the chai to remove the herbs, and add the salt and honey to taste. Froth the drink in a high-speed blender if desired.

TEA: A GREAT WAY TO HYDRATE AND NOURISH YOUR CELLS

I *love* tea! I drink tea every single day. It is incredibly hydrating, it is a great delivery vehicle for supercharged nutrition when you incorporate superherbs, it fills you up, and it keeps your cells healthy and juicy.

My Favorite Teas

Chaga tea is chock-full of nutrients, particularly superoxide dismutase, melanin, polysaccharides, and triterpenes, which scavenge for free radicals, boost immunity, shield the skin from UV damage, and give the skin a healthy golden glow.

Reishi tea relieves tension, boosts the immune system, elevates the spirit, and promotes peace of mind. Plus, it contains polysaccharides that hydrate the skin and balance water in the cells, it reduces skin inflammation, it promotes cell regeneration, and it reduces puffiness and wrinkles.

Nettle tea is nourishing, diuretic, and anti-inflammatory, making it a natural beauty remedy for skin and hair since it clears acne and eczema and provides the hair with deep nourishment, oxygenation, and stimulation by fortifying hair fibers and renewing growth.

Green tea contains L-theanine, a naturally calming amino acid, as well as a wealth of antioxidants that improve complexion, heal blemishes and scars, support elasticity, reduce dark circles and puffy eyes, neutralize free radicals, and prevent skin sagging, sun damage, age spots, fine lines, and wrinkles.

Cat's claw tea is antimicrobial and antifungal, providing tremendous support to the immune system, and it protects and lengthens telomeres, promotes healthy digestion, and replenishes the body's energy stores.

Pau d'arco tea is antimicrobial and antifungal as well, making it effective in treating inflammatory skin conditions, and it promotes intestinal and oral health, supports healthy detoxification, boosts the production of red blood cells as well as immunity, and strengthens sexual vitality.

Chanca piedra tea is specifically protective against oxidative stress and is celebrated as the "liver herb" in TCM. Plus, it combats harmful bacteria without harming helpful bacteria, and it contains phenolic compounds, which support balanced blood sugar.

CELLULAR HYDRATION

You are a water-based life-form. When you were a growing embryo, you consisted of more than 80 percent water, and as a newborn, you were made up of about 74 percent water. Your blood consists of more than 80 percent water, and your brain, 75 percent. Your liver, which is the body's primary filter, consists of an astonishing 96 percent water!

Water contributes to a whole host of critical body functions, including transporting oxygen to the cells, removing waste, digesting food, absorbing and assimilating nutrients, maintaining the body's temperature, burning fat, and keeping tissues nice and juicy. Proper hydration also promotes circulation, improves elimination, helps the body flush toxins more efficiently, deters acne, reduces hair loss (water makes up a quarter of the weight of a hair strand), and even strengthens your cuticles and nails, making them less likely to break or tear.

Water rejuvenates the skin and enhances the complexion too. Our skin is made up of several layers. The protective, outermost layer containing pigments, skin cells, and proteins is called the epidermis. As we age, this layer thins out and our skin starts to look more pale and translucent as the number of pigment-containing cells decrease. The next layer of skin is the dermis, which is made up of blood vessels, nerves, hair follicles, and sweat and oil glands. As we move into our forties and beyond, the dermis loses 20 to 80 percent of its original thickness as the proteins (collagen and elastin) that give it flexibility and strength plummet. The final layer of the skin—the layer under the dermis—contains some hair follicles, blood vessels, and fat and shrinks with age, contributing to the appearance of aging skin.

We can't stop the changes that the skin undergoes as we age, but we can certainly do some things to slow down the process and keep our skin looking younger, longer. Hydration is essential and one of the easiest ways to maintain skin health. In Ayurveda, aging is actually considered a process of dehydration. Water supports the structure of our skin, bolstering each cell to remain plump and juicy, creating radiant skin on the outside. The skin is the last place to receive nutrition from the blood, so exercising regularly can help to increase blood flow, keeping skin looking youthful for a longer period of time. Along with hydrating and exercising, avoid too much sun exposure, which increases wrinkles and contributes to a leathery-looking complexion, and use only pure oils like coconut or jojoba to moisturize.

Not only does hydration support the structure of the skin; it is also essential to the formation of collagen. Chains of collagen molecules are held together by water bridges that are essential to their structure. Without water, collagen molecules become unstable.

The best way to hydrate the skin and cells is to drink water, ideally spring water. Other ways are to consume soups, water-rich fruits and veggies (see page 174), and organic herbal teas. Don't try to hydrate with neon sports drinks, alcohol, sugary sodas, or commercial-brand fruit juices.

Despite knowing that water is an important nutrient for our health and well-being, 75 percent of Americans are dehydrated. Dehydration occurs when water intake is less than water loss. Every day we lose water through urine, breathing, bowel movements, and sweating. Therefore it is vital to replenish the body by staying hydrated and drinking water.

When the body is dehydrated, it cannot operate at an optimal level. Dehydration slows down the metabolic processes as well as limits the body's natural healing capacity. If dehydration becomes chronic, it can cause inflammation in the body, contribute to degenerative diseases, affect kidney function, and lead to muscle damage or constipation.

When the skin loses too much water, the lipid layers flatten out and slacken, and the skin becomes crepe-like. When you pinch dehydrated skin, it wrinkles and sticks together without its usual bounce, and it may take a long time to return to its proper place. It will look dull and can develop a scaly appearance. Fine lines and dark circles become more pronounced under the eyes. Without proper moisture content, cellular development is inhibited, leaving the skin unable to adequately repair itself.

Signs You Aren't Drinking Enough Water

- Increased thirst
- Dry mouth, lips, and/or eyes
- Dry skin

- Fatigue or sleepiness
- Small amounts of urine passed infrequently
- Low volume of urine that is more yellowish than normal
- Headache
- Dizziness
- Muscle cramps
- Cessation of sweating
- Kidney pain

HOW MUCH WATER SHOULD YOU BE DRINKING?

A good guide is to drink one-half of your body weight in ounces of water daily. In other words, if you weigh 150 pounds, you should drink 75 ounces of water each day. If you are an athlete or live in a hot climate, you will need to increase this amount. Similarly, if you consume alcohol, caffeinated beverages, or other diuretic drinks, you will need to replenish more, because even though you are consuming liquids, those particular liquids pull hydration out of the cells.

Drink your water at room temperature. Ayurvedic tradition states that room-temperature water is easier on the digestive system than cold water. Sip water slowly, but continuously, throughout the day rather than gulp it all down in one go. This gives your tissues more time to absorb the hydration, and you won't find yourself needing to run to the bathroom as often.

When you drink good-quality water, your body will notice the difference!

DRINK WATER FIRST THING IN THE MORNING

Every morning when you wake up, the first thing you should do is drink 1 liter (approximately 34 ounces) of fresh pure water on an empty stomach. I drink fresh spring water with a pinch or two of sea salt and charcoal when I am living in Canada; when I am in Hawaii, I drink fresh spring water with sea salt, chunks of citrus fruit, and charcoal.

This single habit could transform your beauty for life. First, it rehydrates your water-starved cells. Second, it flushes your colon of toxins and boosts the detoxification activity of your kidneys. Third, it can boost your metabolism by as much as 24 percent, and it can curb your appetite, both of which support healthy weight-loss efforts.

THE TRUTH ABOUT TAP WATER

Toxins in Your Municipal Water

- Fluoride has been purposefully added to tap water since the 1940s to help reduce tooth decay, yet we now know fluoride is a neurotoxin and endocrine disruptor linked to thyroid and pineal gland damage, lower IQs, ADHD, and more!

- The Environmental Protection Agency (EPA) and the Centers for Disease Control and Prevention (CDC) agree that there are no safe levels of lead exposure for children, yet lead often leaks into drinking water through lead pipes (used in older homes), and even new "lead-free" pipes can still legally contain up to 8 percent lead.

- Boiling, filtering, or chemically treating water may help clear out or kill microorganisms, but it will not remove toxic chemicals, compounds, salts, pharmaceuticals, or metals.

- Polychlorinated biphenyls (PCBs) are highly toxic, especially to children, and were banned in the US in 1977, but because they persist in the environment, they still pollute our drinking water.

- Arsenic is one of the World Health Organization's top ten chemicals of major public health concern. Exposure is linked to cancer, diabetes, heart disease, neurotoxicity, infant mortality, and more. It wasn't until 2001 that the EPA adopted stringent standards to try to eliminate arsenic in water systems, but—surprise—it still often shows up on municipal tap water tests.

- Perchlorate has contaminated so much groundwater that nearly *all* humans now test positive for it. Found in rocket fuel, bleach, and fertilizers, perchlorate is listed by the EPA as a carcinogen and attacks the thyroid and the reproductive and endocrine systems.
- Glyphosate (sold under the brand names Roundup®, No Grow™, Weedmaster® DUO, and dozens of others) causes cancer, yet it is still the world's best-selling herbicide and is used in more than ninety countries on more than one hundred fifty crops. It is currently found everywhere in the food chain, including in drinking water, honey, and human breast milk.

Solutions

- Invest in a whole-house water filtration system as well as point-of-use filters for sinks and showers to filter out as much chlorine, dibutyl phthalate (DBP, a plasticizer), pesticides, and prescription drug residue as possible.
- Drink fresh spring water from a clean, natural source. The earth itself is the best filtration for any water. Spring water is the way nature intended it—and when far away from industrial regions and fracking, spring water is typically free of contaminants and toxins.
- Have your tap water tested by a local water quality lab. Copper and lead are the two most common contaminants, and rather than coming from municipal water supplies, these minerals typically leach into drinking water from building plumbing.
- Be sure to use glass containers for your drinking water whenever possible in order to avoid BPA, BPS, and BPF leaching into your water (see page 195).
- If you are going to buy bottled water, the best choice is spring water in glass bottles. There are a lot of really good companies out there, and most cities have a brand of spring water that can be delivered right to your home in glass.

BOTTLED WATER

Americans consume over 8.6 billion gallons of bottled water a year. Most bottled water comes in polyethylene terephthalate bottles, indicated by "PET," "PETE," or the number "1" on the bottom of the bottle. When exposed to hot temperatures, this plastic can leach chemicals into the water, so make sure you *never* drink your bottle of water after it has been sitting in the car on a hot summer day! The worst bottles on the market are the very thin plastic ones. A machine blows up the bottle and immediately fills it with water, so the newly blown plastic has plenty of opportunity to off-gas into the water, which means you get a good dose of plastic when you drink that water. Even worse, hundreds of pallets of bottled water sit out in the hot sun at most distribution facilities, turning your bottled water into what I like to call "plastic tea."

BPA is a very problematic chemical often found in hard plastics, like watercooler jugs and sports water bottles. A National Institutes of Health (NIH) committee agreed that BPA may cause neurological and behavioral problems in fetuses, infants, and children. A separate NIH-sponsored panel found an even greater risk, saying that adult exposure to BPA likely affects the female reproductive system, the immune system, and the brain.

SPRING WATER: THE BEST WATER EVER

Spring water is structured by the earth in a highly efficient molecular shape for hydration. Compared to the structure of water being forced through a narrow municipal pipe (full of metals), it is as different as night from day. Moreover, the earth has added minerals to the water. Just because water comes from a spring does not mean it is safe to drink, though. Be sure to test your source.

You can add the following to your spring water and take it to the next level: lemon increases hydration and helps purify the blood and supports clear skin; sea salt mineralizes your water; infusing schizandra and goji supports kidney and liver health; and MSM delivers high levels of sulfur for strong nails, hair, and glowing skin.

EAT YOUR WATER

Previous generations acquired a lot of their hydration through fresh fruits and vegetables. When you eat processed foods your body needs more water than normal to digest, process, detoxify, and eliminate. It is a double whammy against your cells, skin, and beauty—because not only are you *not* getting the natural hydration through whole fruits and vegetables; your body actually *needs more water* to deal with processed foods. In addition, fruits and vegetables are absorbed more slowly by the body, which helps you feel full.

Here is a list of beautifying fruits and vegetables with high water content:

- Cucumbers: 96%
- Lettuce: 96%
- Celery: 95%
- Radishes: 95%
- Zucchini: 95%
- Tomatoes: 94%
- Green cabbage: 93%
- Cauliflower: 92%
- Spinach: 92%
- Strawberries: 92%
- Watermelon: 92%
- Broccoli: 91%
- Grapefruit: 91%
- Cantaloupe: 90%

Your health and how you look is highly dependent on proper hydration. Make sure you drink enough water throughout the day. Add lemon, your favorite fruit, or a pinch of sea salt to enhance the beauty benefits. Create a lifelong habit of drinking fresh, delicious spring water whenever possible, and your cells and skin will thank you.

CELLULAR OPTIMIZATION

EPIGENETICS

We all want glowing health. Until just a few decades ago, we thought the genes we inherited at conception were beyond our control, that the genes our parents passed to us predetermined our health. If our parents had thin hair or cellulite or were prone to varicose veins, we would too. The "beauty" behind epigenetics is understanding that we have more control than we thought and that we can influence—or *optimize*—our genes to affect our health and appearance.

Just as we interact with our immediate environment, our cells interact with their immediate environment—our blood. In order for cells to fully develop and do their jobs, they need to grow in a nutrient-rich environment free from toxins. When we eat a diet high in nutrition—as we just talked about in "Cellular Nutrition" (page 144)—plus provide our cells an oxygen-rich environment, gained through proper exercise, then the cells can *only* express health, growth, and vitality, which leads to radiant beauty. When our blood's nutrient level goes down and its toxic load goes up, cells begin to express unwanted characteristics. A diet high in processed foods, heavy metals, oxidized oils, and other contaminants will create a culture medium for cells that express wrinkles, mutations, damage, and low energy.

Epigenetics has been a hot topic in the health world over the past decade. It is the study of how chemical markers on DNA shape gene expression. Epigenetics means "above the gene" and refers to how genes are turned on or off by markers, or tags, on DNA. If a group of cells is grown in a petri dish within a healthy culture medium, they grow normally and properly. If we then place that group of cells into an unhealthy or contaminated solution, the cells immediately begin to exhibit unhealthy properties. This is the essence of epigenetics: genes are expressed through their interaction with their environment.

To put it simply, you are not at the mercy of your genetics but rather can go "above" simple DNA sequencing and replication to enhance cell expression. If your mother has beautiful skin while your father does not, then you can express your mother's genes by making positive lifestyle choices.

STEM CELLS

Have you ever watched a Marvel movie or TV show with the character Wolverine in it? In addition to having really good hair, he has an incredibly cool healing ability: no matter what physically happens to him, his body can rapidly regenerate back into a healthy state. Do you know that you have a very similar superpower within *you* to heal and regenerate your cells? Superheroes unite!

In your bone marrow you have what are called adult stem cells. These master builder cells have chameleon-like properties and can morph into any type of cell the body needs to replace or heal tissues and organs at any given time.

Typically a cell performs only a very specific function within the body. For example, nerve cells (neurons) exist to transmit information throughout the nervous system. They aren't responsible for, say, building muscle or creating skin. To stick with movie analogies, stem cells are like Transformers: they can change themselves to perform any cellular function the body needs them to. While they may not make the awesome sound effects Optimus Prime does as he changes, they *can* travel anywhere in the body and transmute into the type of cell needed in the brain, the kidneys, the heart, the liver, etc., to fix physical or cellular damage, and that *is* incredibly awesome.

To break it down a little further, you have about 150 million stem

---

Blood Cells

You have 25 trillion blood cells flowing through your circulatory system at all times. Every 2 seconds, 2 million of those blood cells die and are replaced by stem cells transforming into blood cells.

---

cells in your bone marrow that are constantly making copies of themselves. The original stem cell remains in the bone marrow while the copy moves into the bloodstream. Some of these copies are involved in the everyday process of renewal, replacing aging cells in muscles, tissues, and blood. You wouldn't live longer than one hour without your stem cells replacing your exhausted cells, because your cells are constantly dying.

If you sustain a trauma or are exposed to any toxins, if you fall and break a bone or get a cut and need to fight off an infection, the damaged organ or tissue sends out a signal that your stem cell copies are attracted to. The stem cell copies travel to the damaged area, migrate into it, and then go through a proliferation process to transform into the type of cell that repairs that specific tissue.

Think about the skin of a newborn baby or a toddler. It's smooth, dewy, unblemished, and draws us in with its sweet glow. Babies have a 100 percent circulation rate of adult stem cells in their blood, which is why their skin is so elastic, their eyes are so bright, and their hair is so shiny.

By the time you're thirty-five, the stem cell release rate from your bone marrow has dropped by 45 percent. At age fifty, your stem cell release rate has dropped to 50 percent. At age sixty-five, your stem cell release rate has dropped by a whopping 90 percent! This leaves you with only 10 percent of your original stem cells circulating through your body to replace your cells, fight disease, and repair tissue and organ damage. Is it any wonder this is the point when people start to heavily complain about "feeling old" and start to rapidly visually age?

If skin youthfulness is due to stem cells replacing aging skin cells, then fueling a continuous release of stem cells is the key to naturally

---

Me, My Mom, and Hulk Hogan in Mexico

At seventy-four years old, my mother was arthritic throughout her whole body. Her hips, knees, and neck were so bad she could barely walk anymore and she was in constant pain. I decided to take her to a stem cell clinic in Guadalajara, Mexico, along with my friend, the legendary wrestler Hulk Hogan.

At the clinic, my mother had her stem cells extracted and reintroduced into her bloodstream. Four hours later, we were at a restaurant getting something to eat when my mom climbed up on a chair, jumped off onto Hulk Hogan's back, and started playfully wrestling with him! I literally couldn't believe what I was seeing! We flew home the next day, and in the airport we had to walk about a mile to get to our terminal. My mother walked the *entire* way, carrying all her own luggage, insisting she was completely fine and she didn't need any help. This was a shocking contrast to just a few days before when I had to push her through the terminal in a wheelchair! Not only did she look twenty years younger after stem cell therapy, but she felt it too.

I had a broken, painful tooth that my dentist swore could only be remedied with extraction because "it's impossible for a tooth to heal itself when it breaks." I too had stem cell therapy at the clinic, and my tooth healed completely. No more broken, painful tooth! Every time I have stem cell injections, I feel younger, stronger, and have more energy and vitality. Based on my own experience, I strongly believe that stem cell therapy is one of the most cutting-edge advances in health and beauty technology today.

reducing wrinkles; increasing skin tone, elasticity, and moisture; and creating that coveted baby skin "glow." Understanding this has led the scientific community to heavily research how to keep stem cells stronger, longer.

Research has shown that one of the easiest ways to support stem cells is with nutrition. We can get on the right path to feeding our stem cells exactly what they need if we think about nutrition in three steps: eliminating foods that overburden the digestive system, detoxifying environmental contaminants, and pairing an organic, plant-based, whole-foods diet with superfoods and superherbs. In addition, exercise and sleep greatly affect the strength and replication abilities of our stem cells (and both will be covered later in the book).

TELOMERES

Jeanne Calment lived to be 122 before passing away in 1997. A woman after my own heart, she claimed the secret to living so long was eating copious amounts of olive oil and raw chocolate in combination with staying active and keeping her stress levels low. This is the way I choose to live my own life, and now, amazingly, science is backing Jeanne and me up as being on the right path to health.

As we discussed, cells are the basic building blocks of all living things, including us, and they contain DNA and chromosomes. At the end of each chromosome are tiny endcaps called telomeres, which determine the life span of cells. Each time cells replicate, the endcaps get a little shorter and the cells age. Shortened telomeres have been linked by scientists to premature aging, cardiovascular disease, type 2 diabetes, Alzheimer's disease, and even cancer. Over time, telomeres get too short, which prompts cells to die. Telomeres are basically like little biological time clocks, ticking down, marking the time we have left on earth.

All the beauty functions of cells operate better with stronger telo-meres. For example, when we are young and our telomeres are full, they synthesize a high volume of collagen for our skin. Young skin is firm and smooth and radiant for this reason. As we age and our telomeres shorten, they prompt less collagen to be made. Older skin is wrinkled, saggy, and lackluster for this reason.

Age spots; graying hair; rigid, split nails—these physical attributes are at the mercy of telomeres. Over time, the cells in skin, hair, and nails (melanocytes) lose their ability to maintain skin tone, hair color, and nail health as the telomeres shorten. Eventually, when all the melanocytes in hair have died, hair becomes pure white. Given the role telomeres play in physical appearance, looking older than your age is a sign your telomeres are aging more rapidly than they should.

There is an exciting body of research into telomere lengthening that involves the activation of an enzyme called telomerase, which is responsible for building the telomere endcaps. By naturally activating telomerase to lengthen the size of your telomeres, you can slow the physical aging process! Imagine having the skin of a twenty-year-old when you are sixty or having your original hair color at seventy? This could actually be possible with telomere technology.

While scientists keep working with telomerase, seeking the prover-bial Fountain of Youth, many studies have shown that we can influ-ence our telomeres by understanding how their length corresponds to our daily habits. The way we live tells our telomeres whether they should speed up cellular aging or slow it down. This means each day we have the opportunity to consciously make positive lifestyle choices to maintain the strength and length of our telomeres. We *can* be the person who ages gracefully and slowly, the one who walks into a room at age seventy-five and hears people murmur, "Wow . . . she looks so *good* for her age!"

Studies have found that eating the right foods and incorporating movement into our lives can have an effect on telomeres in as little as three to four weeks.

The top fourteen plant-based telomere-friendly foods are almonds; avocados; beets; red, purple, and blue berries; broccoli; garlic; grapefruit; kale; olive oil; oranges; red apples; sea vegetables; sweet potatoes; and tomatoes.

Research has conclusively shown that telomeres highly respond to many different types and exertion levels of exercise. Exercise encourages autophagy, the activity in the cells that removes damaged molecules and keeps your cells spick-and-span; plus, it reduces oxidative stress and inflammation.

While all movement will positively affect you, two types of exercise are most noteworthy for increasing telomere length: moderate aerobic exercise performed three times a week for forty-five-minute periods, and high-intensity interval training (HIIT), in which short bursts of activity are alternated with short recovery periods for between four and fifteen minutes.

CONCLUSION

Radiant beauty can be attained by slowing your cellular aging and maintaining your youthfulness through nutrition, protection, hydration, and optimization. Practicing healthy habits can turn the tide of cellular time in your favor, reducing inflammation, oxidation, free radicals, and stress, which hack away at the length of your telomeres and turn on unfavorable genes. Thankfully, you have all the tools to counter this, in order to be beautiful on both the outside and the inside.

Balance Hormones

So many people approach me at my events asking questions about hormones. I started doing a tremendous amount of research on the subject and have come to the firm conclusion that hormones play a critical role in overall health, well-being, and—you guessed it—beauty.

Hormones are the chemical messengers of the endocrine system, which comprises all the glands in the human body. These glands take molecules from the blood and transform them into hormones. Hormones circulate throughout the body until they meet up with the particular receptor they are shaped to activate. These receptors might be in the cells of the brain, the skin, the reproductive organs, the digestive tract, or countless other places in the body.

Hormones govern sleep, growth, puberty, metabolism, fertility, healing, tissue quality, mood, and more. They are what I call the "master switches" and require high-quality nutrients and fats for their formation and function. Even the slightest imbalances in hormone levels can lead to a whole host of problems in the body that can affect your health, how you look, and how you feel.

Hormonal imbalances accelerate sebum production, which triggers acne, dry skin, inflammation and redness, wrinkles and fine lines, and hyperpigmentation. High levels of certain hormones can lead to thickened or brittle, peeling nails. Decreased hormone levels can lead to dry, thinning hair, hair loss, or hair growth in unwanted places, like the chin and neck. Increased hormone levels can cause thinning of the hair strands and loss of hair in random clumping patterns.

Since hormones govern metabolism and mood, elevated or decreased hormone levels can cause mood swings, weight gain (particularly around the abdomen), weight retention, cravings for carbohydrates, and insulin resistance. Hormones can affect your mood either directly or by interfering with your sleep–wake cycle, causing irritability, depression, and anxiety.

When working in concert with one another, hormones can be your best friend and biggest beauty asset, *but* when they become unbalanced, they can be your worst enemy and wreak havoc on your appearance.

In this chapter, we'll explore the ten hormones critical to beauty and what you can do to keep them in balance in your body. These beauty hormones are estrogen, progesterone, testosterone, thyroid, DHEA, oxytocin, endorphins, serotonin, melatonin, and pregnenolone.

ESTROGEN

Estrogen is the feminine hormone. It affects everything from the shape of the waist and bust, to the strength and softness of hair. It determines bone size and weight, and increases fat storage around the hips and thighs, which creates beautiful feminine curves. It influences hair growth, both where and how thick it grows. It improves circulation to the skin and promotes collagen production. Plus, it promotes the production of serotonin and influences the effects of endorphins.

There are three estrogens—estradiol, estriol, and estrone. Estradiol, made from cholesterol, helps the growth and development of the reproductive system and is dominant from puberty through to menopause. Estriol is most produced during pregnancy and is considered the weakest of the three types of estrogen. Estrone is found most commonly after menopause and can be made in fat cells, which has researchers eyeing excess estrone as a possible link to cancer.

Estrogen may be the feminine hormone, but men need it too. In the male body, estrogen is crucial for neuronal connections, both for their formation and maintenance. It also helps maintain male sexual function, healthy weight, and bone mass. The important thing to remember about estrogens, as well as all the hormones, is to keep them balanced so that no single hormone becomes too dominant.

For balancing estrogen: aged/prepared citrus peel, ashwagandha, black cohosh, dong quai, licorice, maca, passionflower, raspberry leaf, rhodiola, schizandra berry, and tea tree essential oil.

PROGESTERONE

Progesterone is hands down the most important sex hormone for women. It is the hormone that keeps women feeling youthful by regulating fertility, pregnancy, menstruation, and sex drive. Estrogen is kept in check by progesterone, so maintaining a healthy weight, cultivating a thick head of hair, radiating acne-free skin, mentally multitasking, and maintaining a blissful mood are all linked to progesterone. The precursor for adrenal hormones, it is strongly influential in keeping up energy levels, contributing to healthy sleep cycles, and working to balance stress within the body. Although progesterone is generally considered to be a female hormone, men do produce a small amount that acts as a precursor to testosterone and counteracts the negative effects of too much estrogen.

For balancing and boosting progesterone: B vitamins, black foods, cruciferous vegetables, evening primrose, maca, progesterone cream, turmeric, valerian, vitex (chaste berry), and supplements rich in zinc.

TESTOSTERONE

Testosterone is the foundation for hefty bone and muscle mass, and it powers the male sex drive. In men, testosterone regulates fat-burning metabolism, helping them maintain a healthy weight, especially in their abdominal region. It also plays a crucial role in mood.

For women, adequate testosterone levels stave off estrogen dominance, maintain a healthy sex drive, and balance mood and energy levels. New research indicates that it may be a reduction in testosterone that causes women to lose muscle tone, gain weight, and experience a decrease in their libido.

In both men and women, testosterone directly affects sebum production for the skin. If testosterone levels are too high, then acne can become an issue. Testosterone is converted to dihydrotestosterone (DHT), which lubricates the skin by controlling the glands that produce sebum. Without DHT, skin becomes dry and flaky.

For boosting testosterone: ashwagandha, cistanche, garlic, ginseng (over eight years old), *Mucuna pruriens,* saw palmetto, tongkat ali, tribulus, and vigorous exercise.

THYROID

This small gland has a big impact on overall health for both men and women. The thyroid is a shield gland that holds a negative charge, which means it acts like a sink for cleaning up positively charged toxins. Because our environment is so toxic, many people are experiencing problems with their thyroid and thyroid hormones. The American Thyroid Association estimates that 20 million Americans have thyroid

Iodine

Iodine is an electron-rich mineral that supports and synthesizes thyroid hormone. Seventy-four percent of adults do not take in enough, and yet without an adequate amount in your system it is impossible to achieve total body health. Iodine can be found in ocean plants like seaweed as well as fish. It is considered by many to be one of the most important minerals for health and metabolism.

Iodine is essential for making thyroid hormone. The thyroid regulates metabolism and energy consumption as well as healthy skin and hair. Not getting enough iodine in your diet can lead to hypothyroidism, which causes substantial weight gain. The recommended dietary allowance for iodine intake is 150 micrograms for adults and 225 for pregnant women.

Over one hundred countries, including the United States, have iodine fortification programs for table salt. If you have wisely switched over to sea salt, be sure to get plenty of seaweed in your diet such as dulse, kelp, and nori. These are great as salad garnishes and snacks. Because we require reliable sources to counterbalance other halogens including toxic chlorine, fluoride (fluorine), and bromine, consider taking a liquid iodine supplement.

conditions, and women are up to eight times more likely than men to develop an issue with their thyroid.

The thyroid is also responsible for producing the majority of the metabolic hormones that control nearly every function in the body. Thyroid hormones regulate metabolism and weight, and work together with all the other hormones, including those most crucial to beauty: estrogen, testosterone, cortisol, and progesterone.

When thyroid hormones are in balance, you feel energized and you look radiant, fresh, and youthful. However, when they are out of balance, nearly all your systems go into a type of free fall. You can experience everything from chronic fatigue to autoimmune diseases to digestive issues to cancer. Thyroid dysfunction can cause feelings of restlessness, irritability, and anxiety, and it can put stress on the heart, the reproductive system, and the brain, leading to irregular heartbeats, irregular menstrual cycles, and difficulty concentrating. Weak thyroid function can also lead to gray hair and hair loss. One of the best ways to keep your thyroid hormone production strong is maintaining sufficient iodine levels.

To support thyroid: ashwagandha, bacopa (brahmi), black walnut, ginger, iodine, and nettle.

DHEA

DHEA has a long technical name—dehydroepiandrosterone—but in the simplest terms, it is a steroidal pre-hormone manufactured by the adrenals. The adrenal glands produce many critical action hormones, including adrenaline, cortisol, and aldosterone. When the adrenals are taxed, they have a harder time producing the precursor hormone pregnenolone, which when low can lead to dark circles under the eyes, patches of dark skin on the face, dry skin, hair loss, and acne.

DHEA is an anti-aging hormone that protects against metabolic disorders by supporting the liver and kidneys and by activating cells to properly metabolize fats and sugars. This has a direct impact on weight and diabetes management. DHEA also promotes sebum and collagen production as well as skin hydration and skin strength. In addition, DHEA is essential for stable moods, an overall sense of well-being, and healthy sexuality throughout late adulthood.

Low levels of DHEA in postmenopausal women and andropausal men can lead to deterioration of the immune system, degradation of muscles, and cognitive dysfunction. Keep your DHEA levels high and your adrenals functioning properly by getting plenty of sleep and eating a diet with adequate levels of omega-3 fatty acids (especially ALA and DHA), including algae, fish, or krill oil (depending on your preference), cold-pressed extra-virgin olive oil, cold-pressed virgin coconut oil, hemp seeds, and pumpkin seeds.

To support nutritional DHEA: cordyceps, DHEA supplements, maca, magnesium, rhodiola, tongkat ali, tribulus, and vitamin C.

OXYTOCIN

Oxytocin, referred to sometimes as the "cuddle hormone," is released during and after childbirth and also when you are making love. Oxytocin creates strong bonds between you and your loved ones, which has a direct effect on your outward appearance. The glow and shine that emanate from a woman's skin and eyes after delivering a baby is a direct result of the release of oxytocin. It has this same effect when released in men and children as well.

It is important to mention that for many women there is a trend of oxytocin deficiency that is seriously affecting the way they feel about their appearance and sexuality. Oxytocin is a bonding hormone, and it increases in women when sharing and communicating. In a society in which people are becoming increasingly isolated from one another, low oxytocin levels can make women feel alone, depressed, unloved, and unattractive. Cultivating a strong network of female friends and family will ensure sufficient oxytocin levels.

ENDORPHINS

Endorphins are essential for feeling pleasure and euphoria. They also relieve pain. They are released during periods of strenuous exercise, increased emotional stress, pain, and orgasm. They directly affect your sense of happiness, your satisfaction with life, and your well-being.

Endorphins are particularly helpful in mitigating the skin-damaging effects of cortisol. Regular stimulation of endorphin receptors ensures younger, dewy skin.

To influence endorphin production: exercise, lavender, and vanilla.

SEROTONIN

Though serotonin is a neurotransmitter, it acts in similar ways to hormones. It is primarily manufactured in the gut, where doses of it are released when you feel important, significant, depressed, or lonely. Not only is serotonin responsible for moderating mood fluctuations; it also supports healthy sleep cycles, boosts the immune system, and regulates the cardiovascular and gastrointestinal systems.

Serotonin provides a significant boost to your mood, which explains the primary reason you may reach for dark chocolate when you're feeling low. Dark chocolate is a rich source of L-tryptophan, which your body converts to serotonin (and melatonin).

Certain serotonin receptors in the human body have been identified in connection with the itch of eczema, psoriasis, and other skin disorders. When serotonin levels are high, skin is healthy and glows naturally from within.

To support serotonin: black foods, exercise, Saint John's wort, tryptophan-rich foods, tryptophan or 5HTP supplements, vitamin D, and zinc supplements.

MELATONIN

Melatonin is an anti-aging hormone that supports the production of collagen and elastin for smooth, glowing skin. It has antioxidant properties that not only protect the skin from sun damage but also serve to repair damaged skin cells. Perhaps the most important contribution that melatonin makes for beauty is its power to regulate the sleep–wake cycle. Beauty sleep is more than just a catnap now and then. (You can read all about how sleep contributes to beauty in the "Natural Hormone Balance and Sleep" section, page 205.)

PREGNENOLONE

From pregnenolone, the body makes every other steroid hormone that it needs to thrive: testosterone, estrogen, progesterone, cortisol, and DHEA. With enough pregnenolone on board, you are adaptable to stress and feel happy even when things don't go your way. When pregnenolone decreases, you can experience sexual decline, a loss of energy, sleep disturbances, weakness, arthritis, and cardiovascular impairment. All of these lead to creaking, cracking, croaking bodies.

To build pregnenolone: coconut, ghee or grass-fed butter, olive oil, and yams.

HORMONE IMBALANCES

Chances are, since you're reading this book, you've recently experienced one of the many signs of hormone imbalance: persistent weight gain, loss of muscle mass, low sex drive, fatigue, brain fog, irritability, poor sleep, sweating, bloating, cravings, hair thinning and loss, hair growth in unwanted places, acne breakouts, mood changes, or others. Hormone imbalances are an epidemic in today's fast-paced, toxin-filled world. So many women and men approach me at my lectures or email me about how they look and feel tired all the time. They are stressed out, have lost their libido, are experiencing brain fog, can't lose weight no matter how much they exercise, and are suffering from cramps, mood swings, and lethargy. I actually had one woman ask me, "Why are women's bodies defective?" Women's bodies aren't flawed! They are perfectly designed. It's our modern lifestyle that has serious problems inherent in it. This is causing us to live unbalanced lives, and hormone imbalances are a result.

All hormones interact with one another. When one hormone gets out of balance, it affects all the others. The common analogy is that hormones are like a symphony. When all the instruments are in tune, playing together, it's melodic and beautiful, but if the drums miss the beat, the music is no longer beautiful.

Based on my research, hormone imbalances are fixable through

Tests That Help You Understand Your Hormones

Here is a list of hormone tests that are helpful, recommended by my friend Dr. Sara Gottfried, author of *Younger* and *The Hormone Reset Diet*.

- Thyroid panel: TSH, free T3, reverse T3
- Adrenal panel: cortisol, DHEA
- Sex hormones: estradiol; progesterone; DHEA; free, bioavailable, and total testosterone
- Liver function: ALT, AST, total bilirubin
- Fasting blood glucose
- Hemoglobin A1c
- Homocysteine
- High-Sensitivity C-Reactive Protein (hs-CRP)
- Leptin
- Insulin
- IGF-1

proper diet, nutrition, exercise, stress management, and simple life-style changes. Conventional medicine would have you believe that mood swings, weight gain, and adult acne are inevitable and unavoidable, and that the only way to solve these problems is through surgery, synthetic hormone replacement, and drugs, drugs, and more drugs!

All of what I am teaching you in this book will enable you to make changes *now* for the better, so ideally you won't ever have to face hormonal imbalances. When your hormones are out of balance, they are crying for help to get you to address the root of the problem, not just mask your symptoms with drugs and over-the-counter remedies.

It is possible to maintain a youthful glow and be filled with vitality, because beauty is easy to achieve when your hormones are in balance. All of my research has led me to three main reasons why so many men and women are struggling with this:

- Estrogen dominance
- Insulin resistance
- Cortisol elevation

We have to get estrogen, insulin, and cortisol back into balance to allow our potential for extraordinary beauty to shine.

ESTROGEN DOMINANCE

Estrogen dominance is the new norm for many people. For men, it shows up as the dreaded beer belly, muscle loss, and a lack of drive. It causes men to become irritable and impossible to live with! If you are wondering what happened to your lean, passionate, driven man, estrogen dominance got him. For women, it is the muffin top, a bloated face, and a drop in sex drive. Even varicose veins can be caused by estrogen dominance. The following are the top estrogen disruptors you need to be aware of:

Xenoestrogens are the deadliest estrogens. Our environment is loaded with these human-made xenoestrogens, which mimic real estrogens and have a devastating impact upon beauty, radiance, and drive. You can find them in food dyes, cosmetics, cleaning products, plastics, mattresses, carpets, herbicides, pesticides, and even the coating on paper receipts!

Parabens are common preservatives and perhaps the foremost chemical group responsible for disrupting the endocrine system; parabens wreak havoc on our sex hormones. Long-chain parabens can mimic estrogens and have been shown, even in low doses, to activate the human epidermal growth factor receptor on cancer genes. A growing body of consumers is demanding that the long-term effects of accumulated parabens in the body be evaluated, as parabens have been found in over 90 percent of human breast cancer tumors studied and are questioned in relation to declining sperm counts in men. On personal care product labels, parabens are often listed with the prefixes ethyl, methyl, propyl, isopropyl, butyl, or isobutyl and can be found in everything from deodorants to toothpastes, soaps and sunscreens, shampoos and conditioners.

Phthalates are a highly toxic family of industrial chemicals added to plastics to make them flexible. Phthalates are particularly pernicious because they vaporize easily, are colorless and odorless, and easily slough off into the environment. They can be absorbed into the body by inhalation, ingestion, or through the skin into the bloodstream. The CDC states that phthalates are detected in nearly every American, from babies to adults. Phthalates are responsible for major thyroid and reproductive system toxicity, manifesting as early onset of puberty in girls, permanent reproductive abnormalities in baby boys, reduced sperm quantity and testosterone in men, decreased thyroid hormones, and asthma problems. What's even more shocking is that phthalates are often hidden in products, as they are, for example, one of the many ingredients that can make up the ingredient "fragrance" in a product. Watch out for cosmetics, deodorants, hair styling products, hand and body lotions, nail polishes, sanitary pads and tampons, and anything containing fragrance.

BPA's endocrine-disrupting toxicity was brought to the attention of the masses when the FDA banned BPA from sippy cups and other baby products. Unfortunately, "BPA-free" doesn't mean safe *or* healthy, as manufacturers have substituted in bisphenol S (BPS) and bisphenol F (BPF), which are just as hormonally disruptive. BPA is still found in too many personal care and plastic products to count—endless amounts of canned goods, take-out boxes, water bottles, and single-cup coffee makers, and every receipt you are handed from a cashier. Count on these endocrine disruptors to block the proper functioning of your metabolic hormones, a problem directly associated with heart disease, diabetes, and obesity. Scientific studies have linked BPA to infertility, breast cancer, sperm abnormalities, and sexual dysfunction in men. Both BPA and BPS have been shown to cross the placenta, affecting the growth of infants in utero.

Volatile organic compounds (VOCs) are nasty gaseous chemicals, such as formaldehyde, styrene, benzene, and trichloroethylene, that are released into the air from almost every front in the home. They can be in the water, which when heated releases them into the air. They permeate the air around upholstery, particleboard furniture, carpets, paints, wallpaper, adhesives, and more. Toxic exposure to VOCs can cause skin lesions, skin yellowing, and defatting of the skin, which leads to skin rashes, skin redness, and scaly dry skin. They disrupt the metabolic hormones so the body does not burn its fuel efficiently and the metabolites are not flushed through and excreted properly. This creates a cascade of aging effects: we become weaker, our skin becomes thinner, we start to go gray, and we lose strength and vitality.

Sunscreen has long been promoted to protect the skin from UV damage from the sun. We're taught to slather on sunscreen from a young age to protect our skin from cancerous melanomas, and yet there is no scientific evidence to back up this claim. As you've read throughout this book, there are many foods you can eat and products you can use to boost your skin's natural defenses against UV damage. I strongly recommend this chemical-free approach, especially in light of the strong evidence that chemical sunscreen ingredients (called UV filters) cause significant hormone disruptions. Not only are the active ingredients disruptive; many of the inactive ingredients in sunscreens, such as phthalates, BPA, synthetic fragrances, and parabens, have been proven to disrupt the endocrine system.

Remember that whether you are male or female, all of your hormones must be in proper balance in order to maintain health and beauty for the long haul. If you are experiencing any of the symptoms of estrogen dominance mentioned earlier or anywhere else in this book, you'll also want to avoid the following high-estrogen food sources:

Unfermented GMO Soy

In the East, soy is grown and prepared traditionally, without genetic engineering and without overprocessing. In fact, most soy eaten in the East has undergone only the natural process of fermentation, a practice that promotes the healthy growth of probiotics that help the body digest food properly.

In contrast, US soybeans have been genetically engineered since

1994. This is an issue that affects not only the health and beauty of men and women; children are also being exposed to more and more of these phytoestrogens on a daily basis. Soy and soy products are used in nearly 60 percent of processed foods found on grocery store shelves, in school cafeterias, and in restaurants all over the United States. US-grown soy is also the most common base for protein powders, protein bars, *and* infant formulas. ·

Soy products contain isoflavones, which are known to disrupt thyroid hormones, leading to hyperthyroidism and goiter. They are also known endocrine-disrupting phytoestrogens (plant-derived estrogens), which attach themselves to estrogen receptors, nudging out true estrogens. They can both mimic estrogen and act exactly opposite to it. Giving infants and young men and women soy is like giving them birth control pills. Phytoestrogens not only affect reproduction but also sexual vitality, growth, hormonal development, and eventually longevity and beauty.

Conventional Meat

The FDA allows the use of steroid hormone implants in beef cattle. This means that the hormones given to cattle include natural estradiol, testosterone, and progesterone as well as several synthetic hormones, which are growth promoters. These hormones stimulate not only growth but also an increase in naturally produced hormones. The levels of these natural hormones, like testosterone, progesterone, and estrogen, can sometimes be as high as seven to twenty times the normal amount.

Most cattle subsist on a high-carb diet heavily contaminated with pesticides and GMOs, then the meat is irradiated before it's sent to grocery stores. Once in grocery stores, beef is sometimes drenched in chlorine to kill bacteria. Furthermore, if the animals are stressed, which they usually are because of overcrowding in feedlots, then we're also eating their elevated stress hormones. This is alarming, particularly because over the past few decades young children with elevated hormones are demonstrating numerous imbalances and negative outcomes relating to puberty, fertility, and sexual development. I strongly urge you to protect yourself and your family if you choose to eat meat by getting to know your local farmer and only procuring grass-fed beef and pasture-raised poultry (because factory-farmed chickens are also fed a diet high in GMO and pesticide-laced grains).

Conventional Dairy Products

Just like with humans, cows produce less milk when it is pumped than when a baby is nursing to stimulate lactation. Therefore cows raised conventionally are typically given medications to improve their milk production. Over twenty different phytoestrogen hormones and medications, including estradiol, have been found in conventional milk.

You've probably seen labels on dairy products stating they are rBGH- or hormone-free. That's a great start, but it's not the only concern with conventionally raised cows. Free-range cows are pregnant just a couple of times a year, and they lactate only until their calves are weaned. In contrast, a typical dairy cow is kept pregnant and/or lactating for most of the year. This really messes with their hormones, and those hormones wind up in your milk products.

In particular, conventional dairy products contain insulin-growth factor and excess estrogen. These lead to blood sugar spikes and mood swings, among other hormonal issues. This excess estrogen may be, in fact, the leading reason girls are starting puberty younger and younger. In 2010, girls were documented to be starting puberty as early as seven and eight years old! The most recent research is pointing directly to environmental exposure to hormones.

Estrogen Dominance Solutions

Nature's answer to estrogen dominance is a compound called diindo-lylmethane (DIM). DIM comes from indole-3-carbinol (I3C), which is found in cruciferous vegetables like broccoli and cabbage. DIM helps the body detoxify bad estrogens and also prevents good estrogens and other helpful hormones, like testosterone, from flipping into bad estrogens. One of the challenges of hormone therapies is this flipping of a good hormone into a bad one, called aromatization. In an estrogen dominant person it is easier for aromatization to occur, but DIM helps block this. DIM is a great indirect fat burner too, through promoting good estrogen metabolites and higher free testosterone. Consuming foods high in DIM, like arugula, broccoli, cabbage, cauliflower, kale, mustard greens, and turnips—and consuming even more than your grandparents did—will help counteract this new threat to your beauty and health.

You can further protect yourself by filtering your drinking water; limiting your exposure to toxins found in clothing and cosmetics and the VOCs described earlier; supplementing with probiotics and glutathione-supporting products; and adding the following SOD- and sulfur-rich, glutathione-supporting, xenobiotic-eliminating foods to your diet (please choose organic!): apples, berries, broccoli, cabbage, cauliflower, garlic, ginger, olives and cold-pressed olive oil, pomegranates, and tomatoes.

INSULIN RESISTANCE

Insulin is a hormone produced by the pancreas that enables the body to transfer energy from the food we eat to our cells in the form of glucose. When we eat food like carbohydrates, a portion of that food is turned into glucose (sugar), which circulates in the blood. When sugar circulates in the blood, insulin is produced. Insulin acts as an escort, bringing glucose to cells to see if they will open a door and let it in.

White flour, sugary foods, and processed foods flood the body with a massive amount of glucose in a very short amount of time. Whenever we load up on low-nutrient carbs, insulin goes into overdrive to present the glucose to the cells. If insulin knocks too much, like a nosy neighbor, then the cells simply don't answer.

So where does the nosy neighbor go when the cells don't answer the door? Insulin cannot let glucose simply stay wandering around in the blood, because glucose needs a home, so the body builds it a home: fat. The liver takes all that unwelcome glucose and does the best it can by turning it into fat. When the body has high levels of insulin—from a carb-rich diet, overeating, or especially eating late at night—it becomes a fat-storing machine. Insulin signals the body to *stop* burning fat and instead store it. So even if you are dieting, when your carbs are too high or you are eating at the wrong time, your body will store fat instead of burn it.

Insulin resistance is a vicious cycle of glucose turning into fat, which further increases insulin resistance and prompts more glucose to store as fat. This is becoming such an epidemic in our society that it is sparking unprecedented levels of obesity and diabetes.

I believe this is important, so I'm going to say it again: *The more insulin your body produces, the harder it is to burn fat.* So here is a simple plan to get your insulin level back to normal. Thankfully, all it requires is some attention to your dietary choices.

Insulin Resistance Solutions

When you eliminate insulin resistance, you can burn fat easily through moderate exercise and diet, just as your body was designed to do. Your liver is freed up to eliminate toxins that pollute the blood and skin, instead of acting as the backup garbage collector for homeless blood glucose. Most important, you have more energy, which makes it easy to remain active because your body is no longer burdened by a never-ending loop of excess insulin, fat production, and hormone imbalance. Without addressing insulin resistance, it is impossible to reach your weight-loss goals.

Let's go through what you should eat in order to support your insulin in a positive way.

Cut out white flour (including bagels, breads, donuts, pasta, pizza), soda, white rice, and processed oils found in chips and snacks.

Add in good carbs (like black or wild rice, most fruits, and all vegetables), good fats (like avocados, chia seeds, coconut, coconut oil, nuts, and olive oil), and vegetable proteins (like beans, broccoli, chickpeas, hemp, kale, quinoa, spinach, and spirulina).

If you are especially worried about insulin resistance, or you fear your body may be on this path, feel free to skip ahead to the One-Week Beauty Jump Start on page 241. There you'll find a week's worth of meals, snacks, and tonics for ideal eating.

The following is also an approach to eating to avoid insulin resistance.

Breakfast: Make sure you have omega-3 and saturated fats, along with a modest amount of fruit. Wait four to five hours before lunch.

Lunch: This meal should be rich in vegetables with a moderate amount of protein and healthy fats.

Snack: Make a trail mix with superfoods like goji, nuts, and seeds.

Dinner: Eat no later than 7 p.m., and the meal should be high in raw vegetables, moderate in protein, and low in fat.

In addition to eating according to these guidelines, add twenty minutes of exercise three days a week.

CORTISOL ELEVATION

We are aging faster than ever, and it's showing in our body shape. Our modern environment, diet, and pace of life have conspired to wreak havoc on our metabolism. More people are gracefully leaving their twenties having maintained a normal metabolism only to be struck in their thirties by a sudden tempest of hormonal imbalance, increased toxicity, and metabolic dysfunction. We expect these symptoms to show up when we reach our fifties or sixties, but now they're arriving two or three decades earlier.

Cortisol is the primary hormone released by our adrenal glands. Its job is to get us moving in the morning, help us sleep soundly at night, and provide us with enough energy to function optimally during the day by balancing fat burning with fat storage.

Cortisol is also associated with the body's fight-or-flight mechanism, which in today's world is the primary culprit of visceral belly fat. When we feel stressed, our adrenal glands produce cortisol to flood our blood with glucose. This gives us immediate access to energy to either "fight" or "fly." Just a few hundred years ago we faced more life-or-death stresses than what we experience today. Wild animals, war, famine, virulent disease, and other threats to our survival warranted spikes in cortisol to keep us alive. In the modern world, we have far more safety and security, yet our bodies are not able to differentiate between today's forms of stress. When we are stressed at work, with family, or even just keeping up with to-do lists, our bodies react as if we are being chased by a wild tiger. Cortisol floods our bodies with glucose in preparation to fight or fly and stores up abdominal fat in preparation for a long time without access to food.

While balancing insulin requires a change in our eating, balancing cortisol requires a change in our lifestyle. The way cortisol regulates the many metabolic functions of the body has evolved over thousands of years, and we need to work with that. Our ancestors lived in perfect sync with the earth's unique and all-powerful rhythm. Their body clocks woke them up when the sun rose, and they went to sleep when the sun set. Sadly, modern life has thrown this delicate rhythm completely out of whack. We stay up late watching screens with blue-spectrum light, we drink vast amounts of coffee to stay awake, we binge eat and yo-yo diet. Stress and frantic activity are now worn as a badge of honor. This chaotic pace causes cortisol to skyrocket, with the side effect of belly fat soon to follow.

Cortisol can age us rapidly; therefore it is a vital beauty hormone and one we must master in order to preserve our youth and appearance. When we understand the lifestyle factors that are throwing our cortisol out of whack, we can counteract them.

Eliminating stress is the number one thing you can do to balance your cortisol. In fact, I believe it is so important to your health and beauty, it is the fifth beauty factor (see the chapter "Overcome Stress," page 213).

Sleep is incredibly important to balance *all* of your hormones, and this is particularly true of cortisol. Prepare for sleep by turning off all electronic devices, and do not fall asleep to the TV or radio. (See the upcoming "Natural Hormone Balance and Sleep" section in this chapter, page 205, for more information.)

YOUR SEX HORMONES

Now that you are aware of how to avoid estrogen dominance, insulin resistance, and cortisol elevation, I need to talk to you about how to maintain your sex hormones. This is the second piece of the hormone beauty puzzle. By both keeping bad estrogens out of the body as well as keeping your sex hormones alive and well, you can ensure your beauty is maintained decade after decade.

When we move into our forties, testosterone and progesterone naturally begin to decline, because nature no longer needs us to find a mate to reproduce our species. Because these two hormones are con-

sidered the "sex hormones," the beauty factors they support, like tight
skin and a slender figure, also decline. This is the start of the slow
process whereby we gain weight and wrinkles, and eventually nature
weeds us out. It is therefore a key strategy to keep our sex hormones
in youthful balance for as long as possible.

Progesterone is the natural counterbalance to estrogen. When
progesterone levels are low, estrogen will naturally begin to increase
in women. In men, when testosterone drops, estrogen will rise. So you
need to boost progesterone if you are a woman and testosterone if you
are a man to keep your estrogen levels balanced.

The interwoven relationship hormones have with one another
means that none of the hormones operate independently. Progesterone is formed using cholesterol and pregnenolone, but when cortisol
is consistently too high due to stress, then pregnenolone levels may be
depleted because it is used to make cortisol as well. Hence the need
to balance estrogen, cortisol, and insulin together with progesterone
and testosterone. It is when these hormones are in their appropriate
proportions that beauty can truly radiate.

Here are a few easy ways to keep your sex hormones pumping:

- Eat foods high in minerals like zinc and magnesium.

- Choose fruits and veggies with high levels of vitamins B_6 and C.

- Enjoy an appropriate daily intake of fiber.

- Exercise regularly.

- Try a simple progesterone cream made from natural, safe ingredients to boost low progesterone. Use as directed: typically fourteen
  days in a row followed by fourteen days off. Even men in their
  sixties to nineties may use this topical cream four to five days in
  a month to maintain health and immunity and counterbalance
  age-related decline in sex hormones.

- Maintain good cholesterol with quality oils like olive and nuts and seeds like chia and hemp in moderation to keep your sex hormones alive and well. Good cholesterol is essential for pregnenolone-to-progesterone conversion.

- Reduce stress.

NATURAL HORMONE BALANCE AND SLEEP

Sleep is as essential to beauty as diet. It is perhaps nature's most powerful beauty treatment. When you sleep, your body is able to repair, rejuvenate, and balance itself on a cellular level. Sleep is essential for regulating metabolism, detoxifying, repairing muscle, and balancing the hormones. Specific regenerative hormones are released while you sleep that are not released when you are awake.

Without proper sleep, hormones become imbalanced, cells build up toxic waste, the immune system becomes sluggish, and you get foggy-brained and grumpy as cellular damage begins to occur. You will tend to feel hungry, and you are more likely to reach for bad carbs, refined sugar, and fried or processed foods. Conversely, with proper sleep, hormones flourish, energy and productivity increase, your body heals and activates many of its beautifying functions, and the mental fog clears, allowing you to make great lifestyle choices and setting the stage for youthful longevity and balanced emotional states.

Although everybody's sleep needs are different (depending on age, lifestyle, overall health, and other factors), it is imperative to get the necessary amount of uninterrupted sleep your body requires. Unfortunately, more than a third of American adults do not get nearly enough sleep. And when they *do* sleep, they often do not get truly nourishing rest. They have trouble falling asleep—so many of their sleep hours are spent tossing and turning or staring at a screen to try to "turn off" their minds.

As a gardener, I watch the cycles of growth, development, and rejuvenation with each season, and they remind me strongly of our sleep–wake cycle. In the spring, every cell in plants is actively building, blooming, and preparing to produce fruit. This is like the morning before we wake, when the body is building hormones to take on the day. In the summer, after plants have prepared to produce fruit by building their cellular structure, they set and ripen their fruit, just like the peak of our activity during the day as we use up energy

Circadian Rhythm

Circadian rhythm is our twenty-four-hour life cycle, developed over millennia from the earth's own cycles of sunrise and sunset. Sleep is not an isolated activity separate from our waking hours. It is part of the overall rhythm of life and is just as important as the time we spend awake. The closer we can get to the earth's circadian rhythm, the healthier we will be.

The time when our circadian rhythm is thrown out of whack also typically happens to be the time when we look our worst. Getting off an airplane after a long flight, pulling an all-nighter, or caring for a new baby goes hand in hand with looking run-down, having circles under the eyes, and being bloated. The challenge we face in Western society is to maintain a circadian rhythm in our days. Our schedules are wild and unpredictable, and we spend more time indoors now than ever before in history. It is vital to our beauty and health to establish a rhythm that harmonizes with the earth's natural rhythms. This is essential to setting a beauty-enhancing sleep cycle. Because I have an intense travel schedule, I focus on spending one measured hour in nature each day no matter where I am. That constant helps tremendously in maintaining balance and rhythm, and I structure my schedule around that one hour.

to accomplish our goals. In the fall, harvest occurs, and preparation begins for resting and repopulating the soil. This is like the evening meal we enjoy before sleep. In the winter, I "put the garden to bed" by cutting all the dead stuff off the plants, cleaning up the debris, and protecting anything that might need support through the cold winter months. Just like I need to put my garden to bed for the winter for rejuvenation and protection, the body needs to be put to sleep at night. While sleeping, the body goes to work repairing tissues, manufacturing proteins, growing muscles, secreting hormones, and healing damaged cells. Sleep also allows the body to perform important cleanup (metabolic) processes that remove waste from its cells.

Sadly, in the US we are trained to think of sleep as optional. Yet we set aside special time to make dinner, exercise, get our work done, chat with friends, watch TV, play video games, and more. In fact, we often write these activities into our calendar, forbidding anything else to encroach upon them. What if we carved out time for sleep in the same way?

If we think of sleep as an essential nutrient—a vitamin called "sleep"—without which our body cannot function, we can begin to prioritize it and protect it. Then we can understand on an experiential level how much sleep benefits us in every aspect of our lives, from hormones to performance, from brain function to weight loss, from beauty to longevity.

SPECIFIC HORMONAL BENEFITS OF SLEEP

When you sleep, your body gets a healthy dose of prolactin, human growth hormone, glucagon, and luteinizing hormone. At the same time, your body reduces the secretion of cortisol and thyroid-stimulating hormones. If you are not getting sufficient sleep, your daytime hormones will circulate at night and your nighttime hormones will circulate during the day. If you fight off sleep during the day, then your body needs to produce even higher levels of cortisol, adrenaline, and epinephrine to keep you going. The following are the specific hormones most affected by and likely to benefit from a good night's sleep.

Ghrelin and **leptin** can be disrupted by even one night of poor sleep. These two hormones help regulate hunger, metabolism, and calorie burning. When you sleep, leptin levels increase, telling your brain you have plenty of energy and there's no need to burn calories or trigger hunger. With a decrease in leptin from sleep deprivation, your brain thinks you don't have enough energy to meet your needs, and it triggers hunger, even if you don't need calories at that time. This results in a constant feeling of hunger along with a general slowdown of your metabolism, which can lead to unwanted weight gain, because your body converts those extra calories into glycogen or fat and stores them in your liver, muscles, and fat cells for future deprivation.

Ghrelin works alongside leptin during sleep. It tells your brain when you need to eat, when your body should stop burning calories, and when your body should store energy as fat. During sleep, levels of ghrelin decrease, since sleep requires less energy than being awake. While sleep deprivation decreases leptin, it increases ghrelin, which signals an energy shortage to the brain. The brain then triggers the body to stop burning calories while at the same time it increases the feeling of hunger. Not only does this result in cravings for higher calorie, sugary foods; it also leads to excess calories converting to glycogen and fat, again leading to weight gain, a decrease in metabolism, and a diversion away from immune function.

Human growth hormone (HGH) promotes a healthy metabolism, improves physical performance, and may even help you live longer by stimulating cellular repair and rejuvenation. Even when you are not growing "taller" your body still needs HGH to repair tissue damage associated with cuts, bumps, and bruises. It is also necessary for healing and strengthening muscles after heavy exertion. HGH is absolutely essential for collagen production. Together with its sister protein keratin, collagen works to give skin its strength, elasticity, and youthfulness.

Unfortunately, as we age, the stressors of life accumulate and block the release and/or absorption of hormones like HGH. While a small amount of HGH is released when you exercise, it is when you sleep that the bulk—75 percent—of this hormone is released in your body. The most important stage of sleep for the release of HGH is the deep-sleep cycle, also known as stage 3 or slow wave sleep. When you get enough sleep (no less than seven straight hours for the average person), you will course through this stage of sleep four to five times each night. For every time that you miss one of these cycles, your level of HGH drops.

HGH has become the latest superstar among anti-aging supplements partially because it activates the growth of muscles. In an anabolic state, you burn more fat, produce more lean muscle, and generate more youthful-looking skin. However, supplementing with HGH has its dangers: it can lead to aromatization and an increase in estrogen levels if you're already hormonally imbalanced. A more effective and safer approach is to use sleep as your natural HGH source.

Luteinizing hormone (LH) is produced in the pituitary gland during sleep. As a gonadotropin, it directly affects the sex organs and hormones in both men and women, and it plays a major role in menstruation. Sleep plays a critical part in modulating LH during menstruation. Healthy deep sleep inhibits the release of LH during the follicular phase of menstruation, while wakefulness stimulates the release of LH. When LH is released too soon or too often in this phase of menstruation, it can impair fertility and reproduction.

CREATE A SLEEP SANCTUARY

Your sleep environment is critically important. You want an environment conducive to the best sleep ever. Your bedroom should be free of clutter, stressful discussions, harsh lighting, loud noises, and electronic pollution. To further ensure optimal rejuvenation, get some fresh air while you sleep.

Many people suffer from all kinds of health disorders because they're inhaling mold spores and dust inside their homes. If you can keep a few windows open just a little bit, even in the middle of winter, the fresh air circulating around your house can be very beneficial. Where I live in Canada, the temperature can drop below zero in the winter, but I still always leave my window open at least a crack!

Ritualize Your Bedtime Routine

- Turn off blue-spectrum lights. Stop using electronics and energy-saving light bulbs ideally two to three hours prior to sleep time, because the blue light interferes with the sleep-inducing hormone melatonin. Instead, try using red-spectrum lights at night before bed.
- Give yourself time to transition. Establish a relaxing nighttime routine to wind down before bed, whether it's reading, drinking a cup of tea, meditating, listening to quiet music, doing some stretching, or just taking some time to do nothing. Your brain likes some transition time between the constant thoughts of the day and the slower rhythms of sleep.
- Keep electronics out of your bedroom; invest in some light-blocking curtains and/or a sound machine if you live in a bright, loud neighborhood; add some plants to your space that are sleep enhancing, like lavender or aloe; rub some lavender essential oil on your pillowcase before you lie down—whatever you can do to create a calm, dark, peaceful environment without distractions will help you get the seven hours of quality sleep you are seeking.
- Turn off your Wi-Fi and put your cell phone on airplane mode to mitigate disruptive radiation waves.

- Ditch your alarm clock. As you sleep, your body moves through ninety-minute sleep cycles. When you force your body to unnaturally awaken during the heavier phase of a sleep cycle, you end up feeling foggy and groggy. In addition, an alarm clock jolts you awake, stimulating the fight-or-flight response and messing with your circadian rhythm, the internal sleep–wake cycle that fuels your body.

LH is no less important for men, in whom it has been closely connected to the proper function of the hypothalamus and pituitary gland, both essential to overall endocrine function. In many places in this book I've discussed the deleterious effects on beauty that endocrine disruptors have. This is also true of sleep deprivation, which is perhaps the most serious and overlooked endocrine disruptor.

Cortisol and **thyroid-stimulating hormone (TSH)** both play a role in wakefulness and energy. I already discussed cortisol and stress (page 201), but I will touch on it again briefly here as it relates to wakefulness and energy.

Cortisol is known as a stress hormone and is often considered bad for the body. In reality, cortisol is a critical hormone and we could not function without it. Cortisol gets you going in the morning, buffers stress, and helps you to perform high levels of physical exercise. Individuals who get enough sleep (no less than seven hours of deep, uninterrupted sleep every night) experience a surge of cortisol upon waking in the morning, particularly if they get out into fresh air and sunlight for a few minutes and drink 1 liter of water each morning. Cortisol wakes the body, signaling the nighttime hormones to go into hibernation and the daytime hormones to become active. As the day progresses, cortisol levels slowly drop, until they reach their lowest levels in the evening. As the lights dim, cortisol goes into hibernation and melatonin comes back on shift to do its calming work. This cycle is not only essential to almost all the hormonal functions in the body; it is also extremely sensitive. Even one night of insufficient sleep can throw everything off for days.

During times of extreme sleep deprivation (remember, a third of Americans suffer from extreme sleep deprivation), cortisol goes into overdrive and the adrenals become fatigued and reach out to the thyroid for help. As sleep deprivation increases, so do the levels of TSH in the blood. Excessive TSH may keep you awake; it also leads to weight gain, dry skin, constipation, and hair loss.

CONCLUSION

In this age of technology when we are tied to our cell phones and when on-demand entertainment is literally at our fingertips, sleep has been sacrificed to the detriment of our health. Being able to work 24/7 has become a badge of honor, and for many people being constantly on the go is a sign of success. We need to rethink our approach to sleep and hold it in as high a regard as we do our social calendar and professional successes. Sleep is a shortcut to health, and many of the health challenges we face today can be diffused with proper nutrition and sleep. Sleep is our body's chance to correct hormone imbalances, recharge our jing, and give us a youthful and radiant glow. Instead of following the trend of the modern masses and sacrificing our sleep, we should adopt the strategy of the ancient yogis and cultures that leveraged sleep for eternal beauty and extended longevity.

Overcome Stress

It is well-documented that chronic stress, which most of us suffer from to a degree, causes rapid aging, makes us gain weight, undermines our immune system, shortens our life span, and can even damage our brain—and from a beauty point of view, it wreaks havoc on our appearance. In addition, if left unchecked, stress undermines our ability to enjoy relationships with others and drastically reduces our quality of life.

Whether you experience a traumatic event, are overloaded with too many stressors at once, or are just trying to manage the day-to-day grind, your body is probably running in emergency fight-or-flight mode. If you're super stressed over an argument with a friend, a work deadline, or a mountain of bills, your body can react just as strongly as if you're facing the threat of a mountain lion. And the more your emergency stress system is activated, the easier it is to trigger and the harder it is to shut off.

When you experience stress, your brain's emotional response center, the amygdala, communicates that you need to either fight or flee. When this happens, the hypothalamus signals the adrenal glands, and they release catecholamines into the bloodstream, hormones that include adrenaline. Adrenaline increases your heart rate and blood pressure. It speeds up your breathing, which delivers extra oxygen to the brain to increase your alertness, while at the same time triggering the release of glucose and fats within your body to provide extra energy. All this happens as fast as you can blink your eyes! As the surge of adrenaline dies down, your hormones respond by releasing cortisol. When you experience chronic stress, this release of cortisol never ends, which causes a plethora of detrimental side effects.

Some experiences generally considered positive are still forms of stress, such as having a baby, going to college, buying a home or a new car, being promoted or retiring, and even—believe it or not—going on vacation! This is because any kind of major change is a direction into the "unknown" and requires you to shift responsibilities and/or adapt.

Stress can also be acute, such as trying to make a deadline. It can be episodic and recurring, such as always rushing to make it to work

---

Stress in Our Society

- Stress is the basic cause of 60 percent of all human illness and disease.
- Three out of four doctor visits are for stress-related ailments.
- Stress increases the risk of heart disease by 40 percent, the risk of a heart attack by 25 percent, and the risk of a stroke by 50 percent.
- Of stressed people, 40 percent overeat or eat unhealthy food.
- Stress-related ailments cost the nation over 300 billion dollars a year in medical bills and loss of productivity. (This is 100 billion dollars *more* than obesity!)
- In the United States, 54 percent of people say stress has a negative impact on their personal and professional life, and/or has caused them to fight with someone close to them.
- Again in the United States, 44 percent feel more stressed today than they did five years ago.

on time or feeling pressure to check social media so you don't miss anything. It can also be chronic, as when you feel totally "burned out" in an unhappy marriage or have a job with demands that never end.

Signs You Are Chronically Stressed

- An inability to focus
- Anxiety or restlessness, with racing thoughts
- Poor judgment
- Memory problems
- Pessimistic attitude
- Easily angered or irritable
- Feelings of loneliness or isolation
- Fatigue or sluggishness
- Low sex drive
- Chronic headaches
- Sleeplessness
- Frequent viral infections
- Persistent constipation or diarrhea
- Chronic aches and pains
- Use of alcohol or drugs to relax

THE NEGATIVE EFFECTS OF STRESS

BEAUTY KILLER

Anxiety and stress have detrimental effects on your organs and your skin. The cell renewal process of skin occurs every twenty-eight days but slows as you age, causing wrinkles and dry, flaky skin. Stress slows this process even further, hastening the visual aging process through weight gain, puffy eyes, fine lines, and rashes or hives.

Cells that produce sebum have receptors for stress hormones. Stress upregulates these cells and causes more sebum to be produced, which when mixed with dead skin cells creates acne. In addition, stress disrupts the ratio of good to bad bacteria in the gut,

STRESS AND GRAY HAIR

The hair dye industry is bigger than the *entire* diet industry. It is estimated that in 2018, the hair care market will gross around 87.73 billion dollars in the US alone.

Over 90 percent of hair dyes are synthetic and loaded with dangerous carcinogens that can be deadly not only for your personal health, but also for the environment. The chemicals in the hair dyes go right through your scalp and into your body, and then the excess gets washed down the drain into our water supply. In addition, all the aluminum foils and plastic bottles used in the coloring process get tossed right into landfills!

The underlying cause for graying hair and decreased melanin production is still a mystery to Western science, but according to Traditional Chinese Medicine, stress is one of the major factors that causes jing leakage. Stress slowly saps your kidneys, which are the lifelong battery pack that maintains your hair color. Stress, drinking, drug abuse, overindulgence in sex, lack of sleep, and other unhealthy lifestyle factors all deplete jing, rapidly aging you and your hair. Stress, combined with all the endocrine-disrupting chemicals dumped into our environment, creates the perfect storm for premature aging and graying.

For over two thousand years, taking jing herbs like he shou wu and rehmannia root has been proven to add more to your kidney energy bank account, which helps maintain your original hair color. With a little digging online, it's pretty easy to find natural DIY treatments for any hair color you may have. Henna and coffee, for example, have been used throughout the centuries to maintain a youthful- and natural-looking head of hair. If you would like to continue going to a salon for your hair care needs, try to find a green salon in your area, and keep an eye on the future of green chemistry, which is working to develop a safe and natural solution for graying hair.

which also leads to acne breakouts. This disruption in the gut affects digestion, preventing the absorption of essential vitamins from food, and this can cause hair loss, gum disease, and brittle fingernails.

RAPID AGING

Chronic stress disables telomerase activity. This prematurely eats away at your telomeres, those endcaps on each strand of DNA that protect your chromosomes. As your telomeres erode, DNA strands become damaged, your cells can't do their jobs, and you age.

A recent study confirmed that women living with daily stress had telomeres shortened by the equivalent of up to *ten years* of life compared to those women who were not dealing with constant stress. This shocking revelation means that living with unremitting stress can not only make you look and feel ten years older but also shorten your life span substantially!

In addition to shortening your telomeres, the continuous release of adrenaline associated with stress can lead to premature degeneration of hearing and eyesight. Recent research has shown that chronic stress may cause a woman's brain to age faster than a man's and may contribute to age-related dementia. Plus, when you are stressed, you don't always take care of yourself very well. You may eat poorly, drink more, exercise less, and/or rely on medication to cope. All of these habits lead to accelerated aging.

COMPROMISED IMMUNE SYSTEM

The immune system is a network of cells, tissues, and organs that work together to defend the body against "foreign" attacks. Ongoing stress severely depresses the immune system and makes you susceptible to illness and disease.

Cortisol and corticosteroids linger in your blood when you are under chronic stress, resulting in lower levels of white blood cells (lymphocytes) and natural killer cells (special cells that kill cancer). Lymphocytes are a major component of the immune system. They signal other immune cells to eliminate invading organisms that may cause disease, and they defend the body against harmful substances. Without these reserves, the body is at increased risk of infection, disease, acute illness, and prolonged healing times.

This also paves the way for viruses or bacteria lying dormant just beneath the skin to be activated and to proliferate, erupting into unsightly and painful skin conditions, such as pimples, acne cysts, herpes, cold sores, hives, rashes, and warts. Around 90 percent of the US population has the herpes simplex virus (HSV), which can generate cold sores, ocular herpes (eye infections), and genital lesions during times of stress.

When the immune system starts to fail from stress, it sends histamine into the body to fight off whatever it thinks is ailing it, which in this case would be anxiety. Since anxiety cannot be eliminated by histamine, the histamine causes hives or rashes to appear, basically forming an allergic reaction to stress.

HORMONE IMBALANCES

Stress increases stress hormones, one of which is cortisol. Your body needs progesterone to keep making cortisol, a process that significantly depletes your progesterone levels over time.

When progesterone is properly balanced, it supports weight loss, a healthy sex drive, strong bones and heart, good energy levels, and increased fertility. It is biologically designed to make you more attractive to the opposite sex in order to encourage survival of the species. Therefore it keeps your skin hydrated by regulating collagen synthesis and reinforcing thick, shiny, healthy hair growth. It also makes you generally "feel better," which causes you to smile more—and what's more attractive than that?

Without enough progesterone, estrogen can become the dominant hormone. Symptoms of estrogen dominance include weight gain, depression, PMS, menstrual cramps, decreased sex drive, bloating, breast swelling and tenderness, mood swings, and thyroid malfunction. Estrogen can also amplify the stress response and even increase sensitivity to stress. Maintaining a healthy estrogen level is critical because it's responsible for the proper function of more than four hundred actions in a woman's body.

In addition to lowering your progesterone, continuous increases in your cortisol level build belly fat and metabolic imbalance along with messing with your sleep cycles. Your leptin and ghrelin go out of balance too, leading to an increase in your appetite, so it's no wonder if you suddenly feel famished when you have a project deadline or are dealing with any other type of major stress.

Sadly, human biology prevents you from bingeing on something healthy, like kale, because high-carb, high-fat foods increase the brain's feel-good dopamine response, so you are instinctively drawn to junk food, like french fries and cookies. It's important to resist the urge to reach for comfort foods because stress eating prompts the body to burn fewer calories from fat and gives you a higher insulin response to all foods.

WEIGHT GAIN

A recent study at Ohio State University demonstrated that even one stressful event experienced within the day before you eat slows down your metabolism and results in your body burning fewer calories, which can cause up to eleven pounds of weight gain in one year!

Research also reveals that even if you usually eat well, exercise, and generally try to take care of your body, when experiencing chronic stress you can not only *not* lose weight but actually put on additional pounds for "no obvious reason."

It's worthwhile to note that as you naturally age, the muscle-building hormone testosterone slows down, decreasing your muscle mass—and so you naturally burn fewer calories. Then, when you're under chronic stress, the ongoing high level of cortisol encourages your body to store visceral fat (the kind of fat that surrounds vital organs) and releases fatty acids into the bloodstream, raising cholesterol and insulin levels. This is when you say hello to heart disease and diabetes.

MOOD DISTURBANCES

When you are constantly under stress, you simply are not your true self. You are irritable, tired, and sometimes overwhelmed with anxiety. Chronic stress can cause mood swings and lead to, or exacerbate, mood disorders such as depression and anxiety, personality changes, and behavioral problems. Even if you're eating the best foods ever, stress and anxiety impede your ability to assimilate beauty nutrition.

The gut—your "second brain"—plays a vital role in your mental health. At some point in your life you no doubt have experienced a "gut instinct" about something or someone. This is because the brain in your gut is made up of 200 to 600 million neurons, arranged in the tissue that lines the gastrointestinal tract. The gut influences your mental and emotional functioning by sending information to your brain, directly affecting things like feelings of stress, anxiety, or sadness as well as memory, decision-making, and learning. Both of your brains are constantly sizing things up, recognizing patterns, reorganizing, and processing multiple scenarios, faster than you can even imagine.

What's really fascinating is that 90 percent of the fibers in the vagus nerve—which runs from your brain stem to your gut—carries information *from* your heart and belly *to* your brain, implying that a large part of your mood originates from those places.

Science also now confirms that stress creates some of the brain changes associated with mood disorders by blocking a gene called neuritin. Neuritin has antidepressant actions, and blocking this gene can cause depression and decrease your ability to adapt to future stressful situations. In addition, continuous depression from stress can actually lead to an atrophy of neurons in the hippocampus, critical for regulating mood and emotion, which can take you down the path to other long-term mood disorders.

Let's face it: being in a bad mood or excessively worrying is not a good look. Constantly furrowing your brow, frowning, or pursing your lips can lead to deeper wrinkles in these areas over time.

LOW LIBIDO

Stress takes a toll on your libido because, as we've discussed, it majorly messes with your hormone levels. A study in the *Journal of Nervous and Mental Disease* showed that stress, separate from mood disturbances and relationship issues, has a direct physical effect on sexual problems.

On an entirely biological level, sex drive is about one thing and one thing only: procreation. When your body feels tired and drained from stress, it doesn't see procreation as a priority. Furthermore, stress contributes to a negative body image. If you feel self-conscious about how you look, it's difficult to get in a sexy mood.

The cortisol level that rises during long periods of stress suppresses the sex hormones. For women, this may mean that they would rather mark things off their to-do list than have sex; for men, the drop in testosterone may leave them lacking a sex drive and even unable to perform should the mood strike them. It's interesting to mention that, should you decide to get frisky while under stress, the act will release endorphins and other hormones that elevate mood—it is a very effective stress reliever!

STRESS-BUSTING SOLUTIONS

It's important to remember that the effects of stress are cumulative, so while all those simple day-to-day stressors in life may seem bearable, they can eventually lead to more serious health issues. We live in the real world, and stress is not something that will ever go away entirely.

However, taking time for yourself, recognizing your patterns when it comes to stressful events, and removing as many stressors from your life as possible are all effective long-term strategies for managing stress. To look and feel your best, here are a few effective steps you can take toward a more healthful way to manage stress.

MOVEMENT

In an increasingly sedentary world, we have forgotten how nature designed our bodies to move! Every day I try to do something, whether I go on a hike, swim in the ocean, bathe in the forest (we will get to that—it isn't as strange as it sounds!), or spend hours gardening. Living an active lifestyle is a major contributor to overall health and well-being on every level and is a great way to de-stress.

Movement increases longevity and energy levels, helps you achieve and maintain a healthy weight, enhances circulation, promotes healthy tissue, reduces stress, builds healthy bones, detoxifies through sweating, boosts memory and concentration, and improves sleep. Emotional balance and mental peace are just as important as what you put on your skin and in your body, and movement can provide and contribute to that as well.

YOGA

My favorite stress-busting yoga pose is Child's Pose (Balasana). Here's how to do it:

- Start by kneeling on the floor. Center your breath, and allow your thoughts to begin to slow down. Draw your awareness inward.

- Touch your big toes together and sit on your heels, then separate your knees to hip width. Sit up straight, and lengthen your spine.

- Exhale and bow forward, laying your torso down on top of your thighs. Your chest should rest between or on top of your thighs. Lower your forehead to the floor. Lay your hands on the floor alongside your torso, palms up, and release the fronts of your shoulders toward the floor. Feel how the weight of your shoulders pulls your shoulder blades wide across your back. Soften and relax your lower back. Release the tension in your shoulders, arms, and neck.

- Hold the pose for thirty seconds or longer. To release, use your hands to gently walk your torso upright. Sit back on your heels.

INVERSIONS

The yogic tradition of inversions helps to relax the adrenal glands, slow cortisol production, and balance the hormones. An inversion is any pose that gets your hips above your heart. The classic inversion that everybody knows is Downward-Facing Dog Pose (Adho Mukha Svanasana). The adrenal glands are what allow us to walk upright.

By lifting your hips above your heart and inverting, you de-stress and allow your adrenals to rejuvenate. It also reverses blood flow and helps to detoxify the body.

Inverting is naturally anti-aging because gravity is the force that ages us. I often sleep in an inverted pose with my hips elevated and legs up on the headboard or against a wall. This technique works wonders when I am traveling and have only a few hours to sleep.

MASSAGE

I am a big advocate of massage. It is hands-on healing that increases oxygen-rich blood flow to nourish your body on a cellular level and prevent cellulite. Massage also aids in detoxification and lymphatic drainage, speeds up muscle recovery, reduces inflammation, and is a great way to relax and release stress and tension, both physically and mentally. My favorite types of massage include Lomi Lomi, Romiromi, Swedish, deep tissue, Rolfing, and Thai.

BREATHING MEDITATION

Meditation is a great way to reduce stress levels and feel at peace and at ease with situations that arise in your life. It can lengthen your telomeres and provide a dramatic boost in human growth hormone, serotonin, and DHEA levels while decreasing cortisol. People who meditate are also able to maintain healthy levels of melatonin by reducing stress and restoring balance. As a result, they sleep more soundly and wake up feeling refreshed each morning.

Ideally, add at least twenty minutes of meditation twice a day to your schedule, but even just five minutes will make a difference. Visual processing takes up about 80 percent of your brain capacity, so as soon as you close your eyes, all that energy can be directed toward calming down, resting, healing, and centering yourself. Here is how to do one of my favorite breathing meditations:

- Lie flat on your back with your heels spread as wide as a yoga mat (or hip width apart). Rest your arms along the sides of your body. Your palms should face upward.

- Place your hands on your abdomen at the base of your rib cage. Close your eyes.

- Breathe in deeply through both nostrils, counting to five. Hold your breath for two to five seconds, then slowly breathe out to a count of five. Repeat this ten to twenty times per session.

Do this breathing exercise once in the morning and once before going to bed. You can also do it any time you start to feel stressed or overwhelmed. You don't need to be lying down for it to be effective!

BE OF SERVICE TO OTHERS

People who help others, such as through volunteering or community work, become more resilient. Helping people who are in situations worse than our own can put our problems into perspective. The more we give, the more resilient and happy we feel.

Enriching the environment is one way I choose to give back. I started a nonprofit called The Fruit Tree Planting Foundation. Our mission is to donate orchards to locations where the harvest will best serve the community for generations, such as public schools, city parks, low-income neighborhoods, Native American reservations, international hunger-relief sites, and animal sanctuaries.

You obviously don't have to start a nonprofit to make a difference, but you can practice daily acts of kindness, like helping someone cross the road or going on a lunch run for your colleagues. When you focus your attention on someone else's well-being, it greatly reduces your own stress levels. Think about how you can help in your community, and get out there and do it!

CREATE COMMUNITY

Social support is essential for maintaining physical and psychological health. It can help provide resilience to stress via its effects on the hypothalamic-pituitary-adrenocortical (HPA) system, the noradrenergic system, and central oxytocin pathways.

You don't need a huge network of friends and family to benefit from social support either. For example, some people enjoy camaraderie among just a handful of people, be they coworkers, neighbors, or friends from their religious institution. And although it may seem counterintuitive, having strong social support can actually make you more able to cope with problems on your own by improving your self-esteem and your sense of autonomy.

FOREST BATHING

Forest bathing (Shinrin-yoku) is more important than ever in the technological world. We spend an inordinate amount of time indoors, and this increases our exposure to toxins and poor-quality air. Spending an hour in the forest reawakens instincts developed in us over thousands of years. We breathe deeper, our cortisol is reduced, and our androgenic hormones increase. These are beauty benefits we all could use!

I forest bathe all the time behind my house in Canada. The forest emits a massive amount of fragrance, which is a chemical signal to the brain to produce neurotransmitters and beneficial hormones. It opens up the diaphragm to allow for deep breathing and helps the body to detoxify via the lungs. It also improves cardiovascular health and blood flow, which makes the skin glow. Ayurvedics say that forest bathing purifies our senses. In an age when we spend a huge amount of time staring at digital screens, eyesight issues, in particular, are hitting people younger than ever. As an added bonus, studies have shown that the phytoncides produced in forest growth boost the immune system. Qing Li, a professor at Nippon Medical School in Tokyo, found that after forest bathing, the immune system responded quicker to viral threats.

Besides the physiological benefits of forest bathing, it is also an opportune time to find wild food and reconnect with what food really is. I have discovered superherbs like reishi and chaga while forest bathing as well as wild asparagus, lettuce, ginseng, and countless others. When we reconnect with real food, we develop a natural interest in growing our own and we start down a profound path to better health and wellness.

TOUCH THE EARTH

I cannot recommend earthing enough. I talked about this in depth earlier in the book (page 161), but it's so critical to reducing stress that it's worth mentioning again here. Studies conducted by my good friend Clint Ober showed a dramatic decrease in nighttime cortisol levels and overall cortisol balance when the body is grounded directly to the earth. The earth's energy not only has a beneficial effect on cortisol and other hormones but also supports a calmer nervous system and a healthy inflammatory response, thus offering effective and natural support for counteracting things like stress and adrenal exhaustion.

I love to be in nature with my feet on the ground. Nature is so simple and pure—I feel like I can really clear my head when I'm out there in it. I hike barefoot and garden barefoot, and when I travel, the first thing I do after getting off the plane is remove my shoes and connect my toes to the earth. Some people have asked me how

I travel around so much and don't get sick. My answer? Earthing.

People have also asked me how I maintain sky-high energy levels with such an intense schedule of lecturing, TV appearances, and book signings. The answer? Earthing. The anti-inflammatory effects of the earth completely obliterate jet lag and keep my body negatively charged at all times so I have energy to spare. Everywhere I go, I make it a habit to get to know the local environment by hiking in it barefoot (and finding natural springs, if I'm lucky!).

UNPLUG AND SPEND SOME QUALITY TIME IN SILENCE

It is important to acknowledge that your central nervous system responds to each and every sound in your environment. It sends hormones coursing through your body, your heartbeat rises and falls, and your blood pressure changes accordingly. All of this can take a toll on your mood and therefore your hormones, affecting the way you look and feel.

Some great ways to create space and silence include the following:

- Turn off the TV when you are not specifically watching something.
- Exercise daily to help clear your mind.
- Meditate daily for at least ten minutes. Schedule this so you don't forget.
- Digitally detox. Commit to an hour per day of turning off all stimulating electronics, including your cell phone. Gradually increase this time, working your way up to one day per week.

TAKE SUPPORTIVE SUPPLEMENTS

Tonic herbs can be used to modulate adrenal secretion and increase the body's ability to respond to stress. Adaptogenic herbs have innate wisdom to respond to the specific needs of your body. These are safe to use because they will not overstimulate the body and will support the natural healing process.

Some of the best choices for tonics and adaptogens include ash-wagandha, chaga, cordyceps, eleuthero, maca, reishi, rhodiola, and schizandra. Other great options are chamomile, green tea, lavender, passionflower, tulsi, and valerian root. Because many of the most helpful herbs grow in extreme conditions, they develop phytonutri-ents that allow them to adapt to heat and cold, altitude, and other difficult conditions. When you consume them, you receive the same benefits and can better deal with external stresses, like the weather, and emotional stresses that occur on a regular basis.

MY FAVORITE ADAPTOGENIC HERB: REISHI

Every night I drink a cup of reishi chaga tea with a little bit of honey in it. It's a powerful combination to reduce stress and build my adaptability to handle whatever gets thrown at my nervous system.

With a two-thousand-year history as the number one shen herb in Tra-ditional Chinese Medicine, reishi mushroom is heralded as one of the tonic herbs, a special class of medicinals so important to overall health and vital-ity they should be consumed every day. Considered the queen of medicinal mushrooms, reishi nourishes the spirit and has been revered for its ability to profoundly calm the nervous system and mind while also reducing stress and inducing a state of relaxed focus.

Like other adaptogens, reishi has the additional ability to balance the endo-crine system and robustly support the hormones, which not only control your body's daily physical functions but also affect your mood, your perception, and how you bond and connect with others. Taking a reishi supplement has been shown to reduce anger and depression, bolstering one's ability to see things in a positive way. In TCM, these emotions are associated with the liver, and studies have shown that reishi has the capacity to increase liver strength.

With reishi being one of the most well-studied mushrooms in history, there is a large body of scientific research proving its antibacterial, antiviral, antioxidant, and anti-inflammatory properties and its aptitude to increase nerve growth factor in cells, especially in the brain. Its unique talent lies in how it gently and steadily brings all glands and organs into alignment over time, which is why it is one anti-aging substance you want to take every single day.

Reishi helps smooth fine lines and wrinkles—as skin is a reflection of organ and blood health. Recent studies show that reishi calms the excess production of melanin, which discolors the skin. Reishi influences blood circulation, which increases hair growth and strength from the root while protecting natural hair color and shine. In addition, gut flora love reishi. By improving the vigor and resilience of gut flora, reishi ensures that the skin receives greater levels of nutrition, boosting collagen and flexibility.

It is important to remember that from an organism's survival point of view, beauty is a last priority. Therefore making sure all the essential functions of the body are in proper order allows beauty to shine forth. If the body is burdened by an endless stream of dysfunctions, it will pull resources from the skin, hair, and other "nonessential" functions to protect itself. Reishi boosts immunity to such an extent and maintains homeostasis with such ease that the body is more than confident to pour energy and resources into smooth, moist skin; lustrous hair; glowing eyes; and a smooth metabolism.

Reishi Cappuccino Tea

8 ounces chaga tea, warm

1 tablespoon coconut oil

1 tablespoon cacao powder

½ teaspoon reishi powder

½ teaspoon he shou wu powder

Cinnamon to taste

Sweetener of choice (I recommend raw organic honey)

Into the prepared chaga tea stir the remaining ingredients, spicing and sweetening the tea to taste. Serve warm.

HOW I PERSONALLY DEAL WITH STRESS

I travel more than three hundred days a year, on average, lecturing and leading health retreats and wild food adventures. Early on I realized I needed a special approach to deal with stress and constant change. Three factors are crucial for me to attend to in keeping my life stress-free: mental approach, lifestyle, and physical and hormonal support with superfoods and superherbs. By focusing on a combination of these three elements in my life, I feel confident I will be completely shielded from stress no matter what life throws at me, and I know this can work for you too.

Your mental approach includes your spiritual outlook. It doesn't matter what your specific spiritual practice may be—any outlook that goes beyond what you ordinarily see and experience and is nonmaterialistic in nature is crucial. I often talk about "doing what you are meant to be doing." There is a saying that for those who resist their destiny, fate will drag them there, and for those who embrace it, they will be carried there. I see in Western culture a resistance to doing what we are clearly meant to be doing and instead getting caught up in doing what will make money or gain public recognition. This is a highly personal subject but one to consider deeply. If you are doing something that you are not meant to be doing, then stress, disappointment, and frustration is inevitable. Even if you are "living your mission," there are hurdles to overcome. Establishing a mental outlook that allows you to deal with adversity, difficult people, and not getting what you want when you want it is essential for bypassing the stress response the body has cultivated over many generations. If you "have to have this job" or "have to have this outcome," then you are setting yourself up for a fight-or-flight response when those things don't happen. Therefore adjusting your mental outlook is the first step.

The earth itself dissolves stress. It does this by imparting negative electrons, which open you up and relax you. This is why gardening is so therapeutic; it has a definitive and measurable effect upon your physiology. Get your hands into soil! Get your hands dirty! Grow what you love.

There are numerous benefits to gardening that go beyond fighting stress. You will reconnect to food and look at nutrition differently. I grow noni, cacao, vanilla, tulsi, lettuce, peppers from South America, *Mucuna pruriens,* jackfruit, and much more. I spend a few weeks each year on my wild garden in Canada. One of my favorite plants to grow is tobacco; the flowers are extraordinary and aromatic. Gardening affects your brain chemistry and is very close to what happens during deep meditation; your cortisol drops and your natural endorphins surge. Gardening also connects you with natural life cycles and the interconnection between plants, animals, and humans. In short, it broadens your understanding of the universe, your place within it, and evolves your consciousness into becoming naturally stress-free. I have failed miserably at growing many different things, but in that journey I have cracked some secret codes of nature, like how to grow and pollinate vanilla! It took me over ten years, and everybody told me it was impossible. There is nothing like the trial-and-success method of gardening.

Another secret stress buster I rely upon is building nerve force. Today, we live in temperature-controlled environments that weaken nerve force. When you are always physically comfortable, you lose nerve force. The body and mind were designed to be challenged—that is how they grow and become stronger. When I'm in Iceland, my friend and I dive into sub-zero-temperature water each day for days on end, and this is one of my favorite retreats of the year. In many different cultures, alternating hot and cold exposure is a protocol for longevity and health (see the section "Lymphatic System," page 126). By allowing the body to adapt to extremes, you develop the ability to also adapt to challenging circumstances that may arise. If you don't have access to a cold body of water, try starting with a cold shower in the morning. I guarantee that if you can take a cold shower every day for one month, then your entire physical and emotional reaction to stress will evolve tenfold! It makes your constitution hardy and your mind strong.

It is worth mentioning that every couple of generations we have to rise to an adaptive challenge as a species. Things go along for a few hundred years and then suddenly there is a great change in the environment—a virus, a movement in the earth itself, or dramatic lifestyle changes. We are currently living in the crux of a dramatic shift for human beings. We have to adjust to the electronics around us, the toxicity, new genetically engineered foods, and countless other changes that have appeared only in the past seventy-five years. Our bodies need time to adapt to these sudden changes, and for those of us who can't adapt fast enough, the results can be rapid cell muta- tions, degenerative diseases, and premature death. In reality, we are asking our bodies to do the impossible: genetically adjust to a radi- cally new environment in the span of one lifetime. This in itself is the ultimate stressor for the body. Therefore we need a comprehensive approach to help the body, which leads us back to the adaptogenic herbs I detailed earlier in this chapter.

Plants that have to live in extreme environments or have to fight vigorously to stay alive have remarkable benefits for our own adapt- ability. In TCM, when a person loses adaptability, that person starts to lose vitality and life force. A measure of our skin health, in particular, will be our adaptogenic capability, because skin is the part of the body that meets the outside environment and interprets it. As I mentioned before, adaptogenic herbs—like ashwagandha, astragalus, and maca—transmit their adaptogenic properties directly to us when we eat them. Regular consumption of these herbs is essential for me with an intense travel schedule and a constantly changing environment. Adaptogenic herbs easily modulate the functions of the body and the immune system, which means if we need to increase the function of our immune system, we easily can, and, conversely, if we need to calm our immune system, we can do that also. Adaptogenic herbs are dual directional, working both ways. As we consume them, we develop resistance to extremes of hot and cold, dry and damp, and other fluctuating environmental conditions without feeling mental or physical discomfort.

Three-Day Beauty Cleanse

Doing a cleanse has enormous health benefits, and it doesn't have to involve radical changes or deprivation or to feel like a punishment! Remember, beauty starts on the inside, so doing a thorough cleansing will help reboot all of your body's systems and can get you back on track, promoting clean eating and healthy habits. You will feel so good after doing this cleanse and will enjoy all the incredible benefits: better sleep, boundless energy, improved digestion, banished bloating, weight loss, glowing skin, and even healthier hair!

This three-day cleanse is designed to aid your body's natural ability to cleanse itself by promoting proper elimination through the colon, kidneys, and skin; stimulating the liver to remove toxins; giving your organs a break by your eating less; improving blood circulation; and nourishing with delicious, nutrient-dense, whole, organic, essential beauty foods. These foods fight everything from sagging skin to break-outs to wrinkles to puffy eyes to brain fog to fatigue. They also are alkaline, anti-inflammatory, and loaded with powerful antioxidants that fight free radicals—as you've already learned, the perfect building blocks for radiant beauty.

The best way to achieve results with this three-day cleanse is to *do it!* I want it to be fun and delicious; therefore different options are offered throughout each day to change things up, so you don't get bored or feel deprived, as well as to cater to individual preferences.

Tips for a Successful Cleanse

- *Eliminate the following foods from your diet:* Processed foods, packaged foods, refined sugars, artificial sweeteners, MSG, soy, trans fats, gluten, alcohol, unhealthy oils, caffeine (if you feel you can, I advise this), dairy, meat, poultry, and ideally GMO and conventionally grown food—I strongly recommend for this cleanse you eat all organic.

- *Mentally prepare for your cleanse:* Remind yourself of *why* you are doing this cleanse and all the benefits you will experience from it. This will help you stay on track, especially during those times when you feel cranky or want to give in to temptation.

- *Have everything you need:* Stock your fridge with the foods you can enjoy and get rid of the foods you need to avoid.

- *Eat mindfully:* Sit with no distractions (yes, that means put away your darn phone!) and enjoy your food, savoring each bite. Make sure to chew it properly—digestion begins in the mouth.

- *Drink lots of spring water:* Proper hydration will help flush out toxins from the body, keep you feeling full, and get you in the habit of drinking more water. Also, charge your water with powerful detoxifiers, like lemon.

- *Dry brush for optimal results:* See "Dry Brushing," page 130, to remind yourself of all the benefits from this very simple practice, which can be done in just a few minutes!

- *Move your body:* Exercise is an important part of any cleansing program. When you move your body, you stimulate your lungs through breathing, your blood and lymph circulates, your liver and lymph nodes start their cleanup processes, your digestion gets stimulated, you sweat out of your skin, your kidneys filter contaminants—basically exercise gets your body going so it can flush all undesired waste, toxins, and fats. Rebounding (jumping on a trampoline) is one of my absolute favorite ways to exercise, especially during a cleanse or detox. It is low impact and excellent for stimulating the body's sewer system, the lymphatic system.

- *Take deep, conscious breaths:* Remember, oxygen is one of the most important nutrients for your body. It helps your body absorb vitamins, minerals, and nutrients more efficiently and can speed up the detoxification process. Deep breathing is also a great way to reduce and eliminate stress, which can affect your overall health and appearance. (See "Breathing Meditation," page 224, for a powerful deep breathing exercise.)

- *Relax:* Take this opportunity to relax by enjoying a bath with essential oils, Epsom salt, neem alcohol tincture, and/or charcoal to further remove toxins from your body. This will help you get a really good night's sleep too! (See "Natural Hormone Balance and Sleep," page 205, for more tips on how to get your beauty sleep on.)

- *Practice gratitude:* Spend some time appreciating and honoring how extraordinary your body is and all the things you are able to do in life because of it.

- *Limit electronics:* This includes phone, computer, and TV exposure.

- *Get support:* Ask a friend to join you on your cleanse. Let people know you are doing a cleanse so they can help you remain accountable.

- *Don't stress!* Do the best you can on this cleanse and don't worry. Take each day one step at a time. You are trying to instill healthy habits that will last a lifetime.

THE THREE-DAY BEAUTY CLEANSE

Choose one item from each of the following sections and enjoy them throughout the day. Make sure to drink plenty of plain spring water in between meals. Feel free to enjoy the Apple Cider Vinegar Beauty Upgrade thirty minutes before any meal at any time of day. For lunch and dinner, prepare one large batch of the recipe on day one, and you will have enough leftover portions to last the remainder of the cleanse.

MORNING TEA

(Drink at least 12 ounces upon rising)

Warm lemon water

Ginger tea

Cinnamon tea

BREAKFAST

Flu Fighter Soup (page 260)

Anti-inflammatory Beauty Broth (page 252)

Digestive Tonic (page 251)

Pineapple Enzyme Flush (page 251)

Electrolyte Lemonade Superhero Cleanser (page 250)

Deluxe Schizandra and Berry Beauty Lemonade (page 250)

Heavy Metal Detox Nutriblast (page 248)

MID-MORNING SNACK

Super Green Juice (page 247)

LUNCH

Mixed Green Salad (page 260), with Immune System Salad Dressing (page 261) or Fat-Busting Vinaigrette (page 261)

MID-AFTERNOON SNACK

Very Veggie Nutriblast (page 248)

½ cup fresh berries (blackberries, blueberries, raspberries, strawberries)

Any amount steamed low-starch vegetables (asparagus, broccoli, brussels sprouts, cauliflower, green beans), drizzled with 1 to 3 teaspoons olive oil

½ cup crudité (carrots, celery, cucumber, cut into sticks), drizzled with apple cider vinegar if desired

PRE-DINNER TONIC

(Enjoy 30 minutes before any meal)

Apple Cider Vinegar Beauty Upgrade (page 252)

DINNER

Fat-Burning Vegetable Soup (page 266)

EVENING SNACK

Restore Your Radiance Pearl Replenisher (page 247)

Chamomile tea

Turmeric tea

Peppermint tea

Chaga tea

Reishi tea

Read this after you complete your three-day cleanse:

Congratulations! You *did* it! You spent three days gifting your body with beautifying foods. Are you loving your renewed sense of energy, vitality, and optimism and your radiant skin? Try to keep going with as many of the healthy eating habits you engaged in during the cleanse. You have momentum now; reverting back to unhealthy eating habits will undo your hard work and prevent you from experiencing long-lasting changes for the better.

Moving forward, keep eating as many alkaline, anti-inflammatory, antioxidant-rich foods as possible. After your cleanse, keep trying new fruits and vegetables—eat as many different colored foods from the rainbow as possible! Plus, eat as many raw foods as possible. Keep the momentum going: eat only high-quality complex carbohydrates (such as sweet potato or taro) and healthy fats, cook with coconut oil, limit dairy consumption, and have fun experimenting with nut milks. Limit your caffeine intake. Try to minimize your alcohol and meat intake. Eat more vegetables than meat. Continue to drink plenty of clean, fresh spring water. Always try to eat organic, and especially avoid the Dirty Dozen (page 36).

Keep up the clean-eating habits you created during the cleanse, and reduce your body's toxic load while nourishing yourself from the inside out. You can avoid premature aging and enjoy flawless skin, a healthy and efficient metabolism, an improved mood, and high energy levels. Nourish your body—don't just entertain your mouth!

Most important, have fun and remember that you are laying the foundation for extraordinary health, beauty, and youthfulness.

Follow the cleanse with the One-Week Beauty Jump Start, coming up next.

One-Week
Beauty Jump Start

Enjoy this delicious One-Week Beauty Jump Start meal plan filled with beauty-enhancing fruits, vegetables, whole grains, proteins, and healthy fats that will keep you energized and hydrated, keep your hormones in balance, and keep your metabolism functioning optimally.

The recipes are easy to make and packed with powerful skin-protecting antioxidant-rich beauty nutrition that will help you experience radiant skin, optimize your hair health, achieve strong, beautiful glossy nails, and look and feel your very best.

Get your glow on from the inside out one meal at a time!

Note: I encourage you to use organic ingredients as much as possible.

	Breakfast	**Lunch**	**Snack**	**Dinner**	**Dessert**
SUNDAY	Chocolate Beauty Bowl (page 253)	Mixed Green Salad (page 260) with Maca Magic Dressing (page 262)	Avokraut Bowl (page 273)	Ambrosia Noodles (page 268)	Rich Gluten-Free Vegan Brownies (page 277)
MONDAY	Chia-licious Pudding (page 278)	Anti-inflammatory Beauty Broth (page 252)	Fiesta Flax Crackers (page 273) with Avocado Salsa (page 275)	Mixed Green Salad (page 260) with Green Tahini Dressing (page 262)	Blue Beauty Ice Cream (page 278)
TUESDAY	Ashitaba Granola (page 256)	Marinated Mushroom Beauty Salad (page 265)	Refrigerator Chocolate Macaroons (page 281)	Fat-Burning Vegetable Soup (page 266)	Raw Chocolate Chip Cookies (page 280)
WEDNESDAY	Energy Bars (page 258)	Raw Burgers (page 269)	Fruit and Nut Super Chocolate Cups (page 282)	Southwest Chopped Salad (page 270)	Easy No-Bake Brownies (page 283)
THURSDAY	Blueberry Coconut Pancakes (page 254)	Fresh from the Garden Soup (page 271)	Herbal Bliss Balls (page 276)	Quinoa with Veggies (page 271) and Spirulina Hemp Dressing (page 263)	Raw Chocolate Pudding (page 284)
FRIDAY	Gluten-Free Granola (page 257)	Avocado Hummus Wrap (page 267)	Very Veggie Nutriblast (page 248)	Mixed Greens with Sweet and Tangy Goldenberry Dressing (page 264)	Chocolate-Covered Strawberries (page 284)
SATURDAY	Gluten-Free Zucchini Chia Muffins (page 255)	Mixed Green Salad (page 260) with Italian Herb Dressing (page 263)	Rockin' Raw Chocolate Smoothie (page 249)	Quinoa with Veggies (page 271) and Ragin' Inflamm-aging Curry (page 272)	Easy Mocha Lovers' Tart (page 285)

Beauty Recipes

You've made it to the recipes! I'm so happy you've arrived. This is the beginning of implementing in your daily life all of the strategies I've recommended in this book. While these are the core recipes needed to participate in the Three-Day Beauty Cleanse and the One-Week Beauty Jump Start, these are not the only recipes in this book. As you've very well noticed, there are tonics, smoothies, juices, and more throughout the chapters. For that reason, I've supplied the following list of all the recipes in the book and where you can find them.

One last thing! As you've seen from my recommendations in every chapter, many of the foods, supplements, vitamins, and minerals that will detox your organs and support and maintain your beauty are not commonplace. You may not have heard of some of them before now. These are typically available at your local natural food store or for delivery from an online retailer. They are not expensive. In fact, purchasing and investing in them will replace your need for processed junk food. For this reason, I've packed my beauty recipes with these healing ingredients. I understand that you may not have them in your cabinets just yet, but I hope you will make the jump toward a more beautiful life by picking them up.

FULL LIST OF BEAUTY DIET RECIPES

Acai Lip Balm (page 53)

Activated Charcoal Mask (page 140)

Ambrosia Noodles (page 268)

Anti-inflammatory Beauty Broth (page 252)

Apple Cider Vinegar Beauty Upgrade (page 252)

Ashitaba Granola (page 256)

Avocado Hummus Wrap (page 267)

Avocado Salsa (page 275)

Avokraut Bowl (page 273)

Bentonite Clay Detoxifying Mask (page 133)

Blue Beauty Ice Cream (page 278)

Blueberry Coconut Pancakes (page 254)

Chia-licious Pudding (page 278)

Chocolate Beauty Bowl (page 253)

Chocolate-Covered Strawberries (page 284)

Clean Sweep Charcoal Lemonade (page 138)

Deluxe Schizandra and Berry Beauty Lemonade (page 250)

Detox Bath (page 125)

Digestive Tonic (page 251)

Easy Mocha Lovers' Tart (page 285)

Easy No-Bake Brownies (page 283)

Electrolyte Lemonade Superhero Cleanser (page 250)

NUTRIBLASTS

Super Green Juice

1 cucumber, peeled

2 cups fresh greens (kale, spinach, chard, lettuce)

3 stalks celery

1 green apple, cored

Small handful of fresh parsley

½ lemon or lime

1-inch piece fresh ginger root

Juice all the ingredients in a vegetable juicer and serve. If using a high-speed blender, strain the fiber out with a cheesecloth and serve.

Restore Your Radiance Pearl Replenisher

12 ounces chamomile tea, warm

1 tablespoon coconut oil

1 teaspoon pearl powder

½ teaspoon *Mucuna pruriens* powder

½ teaspoon vanilla powder

Blend all the ingredients together in a high-speed blender and serve in the evening.

Heavy Metal Detox Nutriblast

Enjoy this drink daily as part of a heavy metal detox program.

1 pink grapefruit

1 cup fresh chopped pineapple

½ cucumber, peeled

½ cup fresh parsley

¼ to ½ cup fresh cilantro

2 tablespoons hemp seeds

1 tablespoon freshly squeezed lemon juice

1 teaspoon chlorella powder or 15 chlorella tablets

1 to 5 pinches of activated charcoal, fulvic acid, and/or zeolites

Pinch of sea salt

Raw organic honey to taste

Peel the grapefruit, leaving the bioflavonoid-rich white pith and seeds intact. Blend all the ingredients together in a high-speed blender until the mixture is smooth.

Very Veggie Nutriblast

½ cup spring water

2 tomatoes

2 stalks celery

1 carrot, peeled or scrubbed

½ medium beet, peeled or scrubbed

½ red bell pepper

½ cucumber, peeled

¼ cup fresh parsley

2 to 3 tablespoons olive oil

2 tablespoons dulse flakes

1 teaspoon freshly squeezed lemon juice

1 teaspoon kelp granules

1 teaspoon ground coriander

¼ teaspoon sea salt

Pinch of ground cayenne

Blend all the ingredients together in a high-speed blender and enjoy!

Rockin' Raw Chocolate Smoothie

2 cups coconut water

2 tablespoons cacao powder

1 tablespoon coconut oil

1 tablespoon mesquite or lucuma powder

1 teaspoon maca powder

¼ teaspoon vanilla powder

Pinch of sea salt

Raw organic honey to taste

1 tablespoon chia seeds (optional)

Blend all the ingredients together in a high-speed blender and enjoy!

TONICS

Electrolyte Lemonade Superhero Cleanser

1.5 liters (approximately 51 ounces) spring water

Juice of 1 lemon (with white pith blended in if possible)

1 to 2 teaspoons MSM powder

1 to 2 teaspoons noni powder

1 to 2 tablespoons raw organic honey

5 to 15 drops liquid zeolite

5 to 15 drops liquid fulvic acid or 1 teaspoon shilajit powder

1 to 2 pinches of sea salt

Hot pepper to taste

Blend all the ingredients together in a high-speed blender and enjoy on an empty stomach.

Deluxe Schizandra and Berry Beauty Lemonade

8 ounces spring water

3-inch piece fresh aloe vera, skin removed

1 whole lemon, peeled

½ cup or more fresh or frozen berries

1 tablespoon goji berries

2 to 3 teaspoons MSM powder

1 teaspoon schizandra powder or 2 squirts schizandra extract

1 teaspoon pearl powder

Stevia or raw organic honey to taste

Pinch of sea salt

4 ounces coconut water kefir (optional)

½ ounce liquid silica (optional)

Blend all the ingredients together in a high-speed blender until the mixture is well combined. Strain it if desired for a smoother texture.

Digestive Tonic

8 ounces spring water

½ cup fresh or frozen chopped pineapple

1 medium lemon, peeled

1 tablespoon raw organic honey

1-inch piece fresh ginger root

Blend all the ingredients together in a high-speed blender until the mixture is well combined and enjoy!

Pineapple Enzyme Flush

For better digestion and weight maintenance.

8 ounces spring water

½ cup fresh or frozen chopped pineapple

1 tablespoon raw organic honey or stevia to taste

1 teaspoon apple cider vinegar

½ teaspoon fresh ginger juice (or a small piece fresh ginger root)

Blend all the ingredients together in a high-speed blender and enjoy!

Anti-inflammatory Beauty Broth

8 ounces vegetable broth, warm

1 carrot, peeled and diced

1 orange, peeled and seeded

1 tablespoon olive oil

1 teaspoon freshly grated ginger root

Pinch of ground nutmeg

Blend all the ingredients together in a high-speed blender until the mixture is well combined and enjoy!

Apple Cider Vinegar Beauty Upgrade

For appetite control, improved digestion, increased metabolism, and high-powered detox support.

12 ounces still or sparkling spring water

¼ cup fresh or frozen berries (your choice)

1 tablespoon apple cider vinegar

1 tablespoon freshly squeezed lemon juice

1 tablespoon raw organic honey or stevia to taste

Dash of liquid silica

½ teaspoon schizandra powder

Blend all the ingredients together in a high-speed blender and enjoy 30 minutes before a meal.

BREAKFAST

Chocolate Beauty Bowl

½ cup uncooked quinoa

½ to 1 cup spring water

1 cup unsweetened coconut milk, plus more for serving

Pinch of Celtic or Icelandic sea salt

2 tablespoons cacao powder

2 tablespoons raw organic honey

½ teaspoon vanilla powder

Hemp seeds and/or cacao nibs for garnish (optional)

Rinse the quinoa in a fine-mesh strainer. Transfer it to a saucepan. Add ½ cup water plus 1 cup of the coconut milk and the salt. Stir to combine the ingredients, and bring the mixture to a boil over high heat, then reduce the heat to low and simmer, uncovered, for about 25 minutes, stirring occasionally, until the quinoa is tender. Add additional liquid if necessary.

Once the liquid is absorbed, remove the pan from heat and stir in the cacao powder, honey, and vanilla powder. Taste and adjust the flavors as needed.

Serve with additional coconut milk and garnish with hemp seeds and/or cacao nibs if desired.

Blueberry Coconut Pancakes

Makes 8 pancakes

1 banana, mashed

2 large eggs

3 tablespoons coconut oil

¼ cup coconut milk

¼ cup coconut flour

3 tablespoons ground chia seeds

2 tablespoons raw organic honey

½ teaspoon baking powder

½ teaspoon vanilla powder

Pinch of Celtic or Icelandic sea salt

½ to 1 cup fresh or frozen blueberries

In a bowl with a hand mixer, mix together the banana, eggs, 2 tablespoons of the coconut oil, coconut milk, coconut flour, chia seeds, honey, baking powder, vanilla powder, and salt until the batter is smooth. With a spoon, stir in blueberries.

In a skillet set over medium-low heat, melt the remaining 1 tablespoon of coconut oil. Ladle the batter with a ¼ cup measure into the skillet. Be patient for each pancake to cook. When you see bubbles on top, flip the pancake to cook on the other side. Serve hot.

Gluten-Free Zucchini Chia Muffins

Makes about 9 muffins

- **1 cup zucchini, shredded and squeezed of excess liquid**
- **1 medium ripe banana, mashed**
- **1 large egg**
- **½ cup nut butter (substitute sunflower butter if you're avoiding nuts)**
- **¼ cup raw organic honey**
- **3 tablespoons ground chia seeds**
- **1 tablespoon maca powder**
- **1 teaspoon vanilla powder**
- **1 teaspoon ground cinnamon**
- **½ teaspoon baking soda**

Preheat the oven to 375°F.

Prepare a muffin pan by coating it with coconut oil or adding cupcake liners. Set the pan aside.

In a bowl or with a mixer, mix all the ingredients until everything is well combined. Pour the batter into the prepared muffin pan, filling each cavity until it is about three-quarters full.

Bake the muffins 20 to 25 minutes, or until the tops are set and a toothpick inserted into the middle of one comes out clean. Allow them to cool in the pan for approximately 10 minutes before removing them.

Store the muffins in an airtight container in the refrigerator for up to a week.

Note: Vegans can substitute dry chia seeds for the egg by using a total of ¼ cup ground chia seeds instead.

Ashitaba Granola

This recipe calls for a food dehydrator.

> **1 cup sprouted and dehydrated buckwheat groats**
>
> **½ cup almonds, soaked overnight and drained**
>
> **4 ounces coconut water**
>
> **½ cup shredded unsweetened coconut**
>
> **¼ cup sunflower seeds**
>
> **¼ cup pumpkin seeds**
>
> **¼ cup goji berries**
>
> **¼ cup raisins**
>
> **¼ cup chia seeds**
>
> **¼ cup sun-dried cane juice crystals or xylitol**
>
> **8 medium dates, pitted and chopped**
>
> **2 teaspoons ground cinnamon**
>
> **2 teaspoons ashitaba powder**
>
> **½ teaspoon ground nutmeg**
>
> **½ teaspoon ground ginger**
>
> **¼ teaspoon vanilla powder**
>
> **¼ teaspoon ground cloves**
>
> **¼ teaspoon sea salt**
>
> **1 teaspoon astragalus powder (optional)**

Preheat a dehydrator to 115°F.

In a bowl, combine all the ingredients until everything is well coated. Spread the mixture evenly on a dehydrator tray and dehydrate it until it is crunchy. Enjoy!

Gluten-Free Granola

Enjoy this for breakfast with your favorite nut milk and fresh berries or as a snack on the go!

- **1 cup raw almonds**
- **1 cup pecans**
- **3 cups gluten-free rolled oats**
- **1 cup shredded unsweetened coconut**
- **1 cup dried cranberries, cherries, or raisins**
- **¼ cup chia seeds**
- **¼ cup raw organic agave inulin powder**
- **1 tablespoon ground cinnamon**
- **1½ teaspoons vanilla powder**
- **1 teaspoon sea salt**
- **6 tablespoons coconut oil, melted**
- **2 tablespoons spring water**
- **¼ to ½ cup raw organic honey or other liquid sweetener (maple syrup, coconut nectar)**

Preheat the oven to 250°F.

Line a baking sheet with parchment paper, and set it aside.

Chop the almonds and pecans, or pulse them in a food processor until they are roughly broken.

In a large bowl, combine the nuts, oats, coconut, dried fruit, chia seeds, agave inulin powder, cinnamon, vanilla powder, and salt, and mix well. Stir in the coconut oil, water, and sweetener. You can start with the smaller amount of sweetener and add more depending on your preference. (Note that the agave inulin powder also adds sweetness, so you may not need much extra sweetener.) Stir until everything is well coated and combined.

Spread the mixture evenly on the parchment-lined baking sheet. Bake the granola approximately 75 to 90 minutes at 250°F, stirring about every 15 to 20 minutes to make sure everything bakes evenly and doesn't get too brown. Remove the granola from the oven and let it cool.

Store the cooled granola in airtight glass jars to preserve its freshness.

Energy Bars

Perfect for breakfast on the go or as a snack in between meals! Make a big batch and keep them on hand when you need replenishment.

Makes 9 bars

- ½ cup chia seeds
- ¼ cup spring water
- 1 cup raw almonds
- 14 medjool dates, pitted
- ½ cup shredded unsweetened coconut
- ½ cup pumpkin seeds
- ½ cup gluten-free rolled oats
- ½ cup raisins
- ¼ cup sunflower seeds
- ¼ cup hemp seeds
- ¼ cup dried cranberries
- ¼ cup dried cherries
- ¼ cup almond butter
- ¼ cup coconut butter
- ¼ cup coconut oil
- ¼ cup raw organic honey
- 1 to 2 scoops vanilla protein powder
- 1 teaspoon sea salt

In a medium bowl, combine the chia seeds with the water. Stir to avoid any clumping, and let the chia seeds sit for 5 to 10 minutes to absorb the liquid and gel up.

In a food processor, chop the almonds briefly so they are slightly ground and crumbly but not oily. Add to the food processor the gelled chia seeds and all the remaining ingredients, and process the mixture until it is a dough-like consistency. If the mixture is not sticking together well, add more water, tablespoon by tablespoon, or more dates.

Press the mixture firmly into an 8 × 8-inch pan. Refrigerate it until the dough is set, then cut it into 9 bars. These bars will keep in the fridge or freezer.

Note: If you don't have everything on the ingredients list, or if you have other favorites, like dried berries or different nuts, feel free to substitute items. The main idea is to get some healthy protein and macronutrients that will give your body fuel for the day.

LUNCH

Flu Fighter Soup

1 cup spring water, warmed

2 tablespoons pumpkin seeds

1 tablespoon non-soy miso

1 small clove garlic

½ to 1 teaspoon freshly grated ginger root

½ avocado, diced

In a high-speed blender or Nutribullet, blend together the warm water, pumpkin seeds, miso, garlic, and ginger until the mixture is smooth.

Place the diced avocado in a soup bowl, then pour the blended mixture on top of it and serve.

Mixed Green Salad

Purchase one bunch each of a variety of different leafy greens, such as lacinato or curly kale, swiss chard, spinach, romaine lettuce, mustard greens (use a small amount), or parsley. Wash the greens, pat them dry, chop the leaves into smaller pieces, and store them in the fridge until you're ready to use them. This way you will have prepared greens for your cleanse as well as for the following days.

You can also make big batches of any of the dressings you prefer (recipes follow) so a complete salad only has to be assembled when you're ready to eat.

Immune System Salad Dressing

6 tablespoons water

6 tablespoons olive oil

2 tablespoons freshly squeezed lemon juice

1 tablespoon raw organic honey

¼ cup pumpkin seeds

1 clove garlic

Small handful of fresh herbs (parsley, cilantro)

¼ teaspoon chlorella powder

Pinch of Celtic or Icelandic sea salt

Blend all the ingredients together in a high-speed blender until the mixture is smooth. Pour the dressing over your choice of greens.

Fat-Busting Vinaigrette

6 ounces spring water

2 tablespoons coconut oil, melted

1 tablespoon apple cider vinegar

1 tablespoon freshly squeezed lemon juice

1 tablespoon freshly chopped parsley

1 clove garlic

1 teaspoon ground mustard

Small pinch of ground cayenne

Blend all the ingredients together in a high-speed blender until the mixture is smooth. Pour the dressing over your choice of greens.

Maca Magic Dressing

½ cup olive oil

6 tablespoons freshly squeezed lemon juice

4 tablespoons raw tahini

2 tablespoons spring water

2 cloves garlic

1 tablespoon maca powder

1 teaspoon raw organic honey or maple syrup

½ teaspoon good-quality sea salt

Blend all the ingredients together in a high-speed blender until the mixture is smooth. Pour the dressing over your choice of greens.

Green Tahini Dressing

1 cup spring water

½ cup raw tahini

½ cup fresh spinach

¼ cup fresh parsley

2 tablespoons freshly squeezed lemon juice

2 tablespoons wheat-free tamari

1 tablespoon raw organic honey

2 teaspoons freshly grated ginger root

2 cloves garlic

Blend all the ingredients in a high-speed blender until the mixture is smooth. Pour the dressing over your choice of greens or store it in a sealed glass jar in the refrigerator for up to one week.

Italian Herb Dressing

¼ cup olive oil

¼ cup flaxseed oil

¼ cup spring water

3 tablespoons freshly squeezed lemon juice

2 teaspoons coconut nectar or raw organic honey

1 teaspoon freshly crushed garlic

1 teaspoon dried Italian seasoning (basil, rosemary, oregano, and thyme)

1 teaspoon onion powder

⅛ teaspoon ground mustard

½ teaspoon Himalayan crystal salt

Blend all the ingredients in a high-speed blender until the mixture is smooth. Alternatively, whisk all the ingredients together in a bowl. Store the dressing in a sealed glass jar in the refrigerator for up to four days.

Spirulina Hemp Dressing

1 cup fresh cilantro leaves

½ cup spring water

½ cup olive oil

¼ cup hemp seeds

3 tablespoons freshly squeezed lemon juice

1 tablespoon apple cider vinegar

1 tablespoon wheat-free tamari

½ tablespoon spirulina

1 teaspoon coconut nectar

½ teaspoon freshly grated ginger root
¼ teaspoon Celtic sea salt

Blend all the ingredients in a high-speed blender until the mixture is smooth, and enjoy the dressing on raw greens, steamed vegetables, quinoa, or anything your heart desires!

Mixed Greens with Sweet and Tangy Goldenberry Dressing

For the dressing

½ cup dried goldenberries
Spring water, for soaking and to adjust consistency
½ cup olive oil
¼ cup raw organic honey
2 tablespoons apple cider vinegar
2 teaspoons Dijon mustard
½ teaspoon Celtic sea salt

For the salad

1 head romaine lettuce or bunch of spinach or mixed greens
4 to 12 fresh strawberries, sliced

Soak the goldenberries in spring water to soften them, then drain the soak water (or use it in a smoothie).

In a high-speed blender, blend the softened goldenberries, olive oil, honey, vinegar, mustard, and salt until the dressing is well combined. There will probably be some chunks of goldenberries, and that is okay. Add spring water if needed to reach your desired consistency.

In a bowl, toss the greens with the strawberries and the dressing until everything is coated, then serve.

Marinated Mushroom Beauty Salad

For the marinade

> **2 tablespoons tamari**
>
> **2 tablespoons olive oil**
>
> **2 tablespoons freshly squeezed lemon juice**
>
> **1 tablespoon freshly chopped parsley**
>
> **1 teaspoon raw organic honey**
>
> **Pinch of sea salt**

For the salad

> **3 large portobello mushrooms, sliced**
>
> **Mixed greens**
>
> **Cherry tomatoes to taste**
>
> **Avocado chunks to taste**
>
> **Pine nuts to taste**

In a bowl, combine the tamari, olive oil, lemon juice, parsley, honey, and salt.

Add the mushrooms to the mixture and let marinate at room temperature for a couple of hours.

Toss together the mixed greens, tomatoes, avocado, and pine nuts with the mushrooms and marinade, and enjoy the salad immediately.

The marinade will store well in the fridge for several days.

Fat-Burning Vegetable Soup

You may wish to add pepper to this soup (cayenne, chili pepper, red bell pepper, etc.). If you can take the heat, hot peppers can speed up your metabolism and subdue your cravings. Spices are a great way to heat things up too, and when you heat things up, you burn more calories!

Makes about 12 cups

½ red onion, diced

1 to 3 cloves garlic, or to taste, chopped

1 to 2 tablespoons coconut oil

64 ounces vegetable broth or a combination of 32 ounces broth and 32 ounces water

28 ounces diced tomatoes

½ head green cabbage, chopped

3 to 4 medium carrots, peeled and chopped

3 to 4 stalks celery, diced

1 sweet or hot pepper of your choice (optional)

4 teaspoons dried Italian seasoning (basil, rosemary, oregano, and thyme)

1 to 2 teaspoons freshly grated ginger root

Pinch of ground black pepper

1 to 2 tablespoons chopped fresh parsley

In a large saucepan, sauté the onion and garlic in the coconut oil over medium heat until they are soft. Add the broth, tomatoes, cabbage, carrots, celery, optional pepper, Italian seasoning, ginger, and black pepper. Bring the mixture to a boil, then reduce the heat and simmer the soup for 20 to 30 minutes, or until the vegetables are just turning soft. Add the parsley in the final few minutes of cooking, and adjust the seasoning as desired.

Note: Most grocers will cut a whole cabbage in half if you ask them to so you won't have any waste when purchasing ingredients.

Avocado Hummus Wrap

2 collard leaves

½ cup hummus

½ cucumber, peeled and sliced into thin strips

1 to 2 carrots, peeled and sliced into thin strips

½ cup zucchini, sliced into thin strips

1 avocado, peeled, pitted, and sliced

½ to 1 cup baby spinach leaves

Sprouts or microgreens to taste

Wash and dry the collard leaves. Using a paring knife, cut off the stems at the end of the leaf area. Where the stem divides the leaf, roll the side of a glass along it to break down the fibers and make the whole leaf easier to fold.

Place each leaf on a flat surface, and spread half the hummus on each near the top and middle of the leaf. Layer each leaf with the remaining ingredients, half each of the cucumber, carrots, zucchini, avocado, spinach, and sprouts or microgreens. Wrap each leaf like a burrito, cut each roll in half, and enjoy.

DINNER

Ambrosia Noodles

2 cups tightly packed fresh basil leaves

½ cup fresh parsley leaves

¼ cup pine nuts

1 teaspoon crushed garlic

1 teaspoon nutritional yeast

2 teaspoons light miso

3 to 4 tablespoons olive oil

½ teaspoon Celtic sea salt

12 ounces kelp noodles

1 avocado, peeled, pitted, and diced

1 to 2 roma tomatoes, diced

Sun-dried tomatoes to taste

Olives, pitted and cut in half, to taste

Handful of fresh baby spinach

Combine the basil, parsley, pine nuts, garlic, yeast, miso, olive oil, and salt in a food processor fitted with an S blade. Process into a pesto until your desired consistency is achieved, but do not overprocess it or the mixture will become too oily. Set the pesto aside.

Cover the kelp noodles in warm filtered water and soak for 5 to 10 minutes. Drain the noodles and then cut them into manageable lengths.

In a serving bowl, using ¾ cup pesto per 12 ounces kelp noodles, toss the noodles with the pesto along with the avocado, tomatoes, sun-dried tomatoes, and olives until everything is well coated with pesto. Add and toss the spinach leaves last. Serve immediately.

Raw Burgers

This recipe calls for a food dehydrator.

Makes 4 to 6 medium-size burgers

- ½ cup Brazil nuts
- ½ cup raw almonds
- 1 cup shredded zucchini
- ½ cup shredded carrots
- 1 stalk celery, diced small
- 3 tablespoons tomato paste
- Handful of freshly chopped parsley
- ¼ cup ground flaxseed meal
- 1 tablespoon Dijon mustard
- 2 teaspoons dried Italian seasoning (basil, rosemary, oregano, and thyme)
- 1 teaspoon onion powder
- ⅛ teaspoon ground cayenne
- ¾ teaspoon sea salt

Preheat a dehydrator to 115°F.

Process the Brazil nuts and almonds in a food processor until they are finely ground but not oily. Transfer the nuts to a large bowl.

In the same food processor, process the zucchini and carrots for just a few seconds to make smaller pieces without pureeing them. You should still be able to identify the pieces.

Add the vegetables to the bowl of nuts along with the diced celery, tomato paste, parsley, flaxseed meal, mustard, Italian seasoning, onion powder, cayenne, and salt. Stir the mixture until it is well combined.

With the help of an ice cream scoop, form uniform burger-size patties. Dehydrate the patties in the preheated dehydrator for about 4 to 5 hours, then flip them over and dehydrate them for another 4 to 5 hours. The texture should be like a hamburger, and they should not be dried to the point of crispiness.

These store well in the refrigerator or freezer.

Southwest Chopped Salad

For the salad

> 1 large head romaine lettuce, chopped
>
> 1 cup cooked black beans, rinsed and drained
>
> 1 large orange or red bell pepper, diced
>
> 1 pint cherry tomatoes
>
> 1 cup frozen corn, thawed
>
> 4 green onions, chopped
>
> ¼ cup sliced black olives

For the dressing

> 1 cup loosely packed fresh cilantro, roughly chopped
>
> 1 large avocado, peeled and pitted
>
> 1 to 2 cloves garlic
>
> ¼ cup olive oil
>
> Juice of 1 lime
>
> 1 teaspoon apple cider vinegar
>
> ⅛ teaspoon sea salt
>
> Water as needed for consistency (optional)

Combine all the salad ingredients together in a large bowl.

Puree all the dressing ingredients in a high-speed blender until the mixture is smooth. Taste and adjust the seasonings if necessary.

Toss the salad with the dressing and serve.

Quinoa with Veggies

1 cup uncooked quinoa

1 to 2 tablespoons coconut oil

2 to 3 cups vegetable broth or stock

¼ teaspoon sea salt

2 to 3 cups chopped broccoli and/or cauliflower

1 teaspoon minced garlic

Spirulina Hemp Dressing (page 263)

Rinse the quinoa in a fine-mesh strainer and set it aside.

Warm the coconut oil in a medium to large saucepan set over medium-low heat. Add the quinoa, broth, and salt, then let the quinoa cook as instructed on the quinoa package. About 10 minutes before the quinoa will be ready, add the chopped vegetables to the saucepan so they simmer with the quinoa.

When the quinoa is ready, fluff it with a fork, add the garlic, and transfer the mixture to a bowl. Serve topped with Spirulina Hemp Dressing.

Fresh from the Garden Soup

Serves 2

¼ cup pumpkin seeds (reserve 2 tablespoons for garnish)

2 cups leafy green kale, de-stemmed and chopped

1 orange, peeled and seeded

½ to 1 apple, cored

½ medium cucumber, peeled

½ avocado, peeled and pitted

¾ cup spring water

¼ cup fresh cilantro or parsley leaves

2 tablespoons miso paste

Juice of ½ lemon

2 cloves garlic

1 teaspoon dulse flakes

Pinch of ground cayenne

Reserve 2 tablespoons of the pumpkin seeds for a garnish, then put the remaining quantity, along with all the remaining ingredients, into a high-speed blender. Blend the mixture until it's smooth.

Divide the soup between two bowls and serve immediately with a garnish of 1 tablespoon pumpkin seeds on each serving.

Ragin' Inflamm-aging Curry

This living curry sauce is raw and probiotic, and can be used as either a dip, a dressing, or a sauce, even with cooked foods, such as Quinoa with Veggies (page 271). Prepare the veggies, then top them with a handful of raw cashews and this curry sauce.

½ cup plain coconut yogurt

1 tablespoon olive oil

2 teaspoons raw organic honey

½ teaspoon ground turmeric

½ teaspoon ground ginger

¼ teaspoon mustard seeds

¼ teaspoon ground cumin

¼ teaspoon ground coriander

⅛ teaspoon ashwagandha powder

⅛ teaspoon Celtic sea salt

⅛ teaspoon pepper

2 tablespoons chlorella powder (optional)

Blend all the ingredients in a high-speed blender or food processor until the mixture is smooth. Use as desired.

SNACKS

Avokraut Bowl

The combination of textures and flavors in this dish is amazing!

1 small to medium avocado, peeled, pitted, and diced
½ cup unpasteurized sauerkraut
Pinch of Celtic or Icelandic sea salt

Place the avocado in a bowl. Top it with the sauerkraut and salt and enjoy!

Fiesta Flax Crackers

This recipe calls for a dehydrating tool called a Teflex sheet, or dehydrator sheet. These come in handy, but you can also substitute silicone sheets.

2 red bell peppers, cored and seeded
1 jalapeño, stemmed and seeded
1 cup fresh cilantro leaves
4 cups flaxseeds
½ cup chia seeds
½ cup wheat-free tamari or nama shoyu
1 cup freshly squeezed lime juice
1 tablespoon Mexican spice blend
2 teaspoons sea salt
Avocado Salsa (page 275)

In a food processor fitted with an S blade, process together the red peppers, jalapeño, and cilantro briefly until they are finely chopped but not pureed. You want to be able to see individual pieces.

In a large bowl, combine the processed vegetables with the flaxseeds, chia seeds, tamari or nama shoyu, lime juice, Mexican spices, and salt. Add enough water to make the mixture spreadable, similar to the consistency of a thick pancake batter.

On a Teflex or similar dehydrator sheet, spread the batter with a spatula to about a ¼-inch thickness. Score the surface in the size of crackers as you prefer.

Dehydrate the batter overnight or until the cracker is firm enough to be flipped over. Remove the dehydrator sheet, and dehydrate the cracker on the other side until it is crispy, about 12 to 24 additional hours. Break or cut the cracker along the scored lines.

Serve with Avocado Salsa (see facing page).

Avocado Salsa

2 roma tomatoes, finely diced

1 avocado, peeled, pitted, and finely diced

½ cup peeled, seeded, and finely diced cucumber

¼ cup finely diced red pepper

¼ cup chopped and packed cilantro or parsley leaves

1 green onion, thinly sliced

½ red jalapeño pepper, stemmed, seeded, and minced

2 tablespoons finely diced red onion

2 to 3 teaspoons freshly squeezed lime juice

1 clove garlic, finely minced

¼ teaspoon sea salt

Ground black pepper to taste

½ cup chopped pineapple (optional)

Combine all the ingredients in a large glass bowl and stir to make sure everything is well coated. Store the salsa in an airtight container in the refrigerator for up to 12 hours for the flavors to infuse.

DESSERT

Herbal Bliss Balls

Boost your immunity and mental bliss!

½ cup almonds

½ cup walnuts

2 dates, pitted

2 tablespoons cacao powder

2 tablespoons coconut oil

2 tablespoons banana flakes

1 teaspoon astragalus powder

1 teaspoon *Mucuna pruriens* powder

¼ teaspoon ground cinnamon

1 to 2 tablespoons cacao nibs

Blend together in a high-speed blender the almonds, walnuts, dates, cacao powder, coconut oil, banana flakes, astragalus, Mucuna pruriens, and cinnamon. Process the mixture until it is smooth but not oily. Stir in the cacao nibs by hand.

Shape the batter into balls or spread it into a small baking dish, like fudge. Chill the treats in the refrigerator to set them. If you spread it in a baking dish, cut it into squares to serve.

Rich Gluten-Free Vegan Brownies

1 small banana, mashed

6 tablespoons ground chia seeds

¾ cup cacao powder

⅔ cup quinoa flour

½ cup sun-dried cane juice crystals

½ cup birch tree xylitol

½ teaspoon baking soda

½ teaspoon baking powder

¾ teaspoon sea salt

⅓ cup coconut oil, melted

2 to 3 tablespoons water

½ cup raw chocolate chips (optional)

Preheat the oven to 350°F.

Combine all the ingredients together in a bowl, but set aside the optional chocolate chips if you are including them. Add just enough water to make a nice batter consistency. Then stir in the chocolate chips, if desired, for extra richness.

Spread the batter in an oiled 8 × 8-inch baking dish. Bake the brownies approximately 30 minutes, or until a toothpick inserted in the center comes out clean.

Note: For a sugar-free version, omit the sun-dried cane juice crystals and increase the birch tree xylitol to 1 cup.

Chia-licious Pudding

½ cup chia seeds

1½ cups coconut water

1 cup thick coconut milk (made from blending coconut meat
with just a little coconut water)

¼ cup sun-dried cane juice crystals or xylitol

1 teaspoon ground cinnamon

½ teaspoon vanilla powder

Pinch of sea salt

In a medium bowl, combine the chia seeds with the coconut water. Stir to avoid any clumping, and let the chia seeds sit for 20 minutes to absorb the liquid and gel up.

In a high-speed blender, blend the coconut milk, cane juice crystals, cinnamon, vanilla powder, and salt until the mixture is uniform in consistency. Add this to the coconut water and chia seed mixture, and stir to combine.

Place the bowl in the refrigerator to allow the pudding to set. Serve it with fresh berries and/or cacao nibs. The pudding stores well in the fridge for one week.

Blue Beauty Ice Cream

Potent blue butterfly pea powder is known to promote vitality and healthy aging. It is chock-full of antioxidants, including proanthocyanidin (which supports skin collagen and elasticity) and anthocyanin (which supports hair and eye health), both of which promote the overall healthy life cycle of your cells. The powder is a notable nerve tonic, and provides support to the digestive, circulatory, and central nervous systems. It has long been used in Ayurvedic traditions to support memory, balanced mood, and a healthy immune system.

> **2 medium to large ripe bananas, cut into chunks and frozen**
> **1 cup frozen blueberries**
> **1 small to medium avocado, peeled and pitted**
> **2 tablespoons coconut milk**
> **1 teaspoon blue butterfly pea powder**
> **½ teaspoon vanilla powder**
> **Pinch of Celtic or Icelandic sea salt**
> **Cacao nibs or goji berries for garnish (optional)**

Blend together all the ingredients, except the optional garnish, in a high-speed blender or food processor. It's important to use frozen ingredients, which means you may have to scrape down the sides of the container you are using a couple of times until everything is smooth and creamy, and don't add too much liquid or you will end up with a smoothie instead of ice cream.

Serve immediately. If you like, garnish the ice cream with cacao nibs or goji berries for additional beauty benefits.

You can store any remaining ice cream in the freezer in an airtight container for up to a week. Leave it to thaw slightly for a few minutes before serving.

Raw Chocolate Chip Cookies

This cookie dough is safe to eat raw! You can also be imaginative and stir in extras, like chopped dried fruit, chopped nuts—anything you like.

- **1 cup raw oat groats, soaked and drained, or 1 cup oat flour**
- **1¾ cups raw cashews**
- **3 tablespoons raisins**
- **¼ cup coconut nectar, raw organic honey, or maple syrup**
- **¼ cup coconut oil**
- **1 teaspoon vanilla powder**
- **¼ teaspoon ground cinnamon**
- **Pinch of good-quality sea salt**
- **¼ cup raw chocolate chips**

If you are using soaked oat groats, drain and rinse the oats and add them to a food processor along with the cashews. Grind up the raw cashews and oats until you have a fine flour. If you are using oat flour, process the cashews before adding the flour.

Add to the food processor the raisins, coconut nectar, coconut oil, vanilla powder, cinnamon, and salt. Process the mixture until it is well combined but still a bit chunky. When the dough forms a big ball, stop processing, transfer the dough to a bowl, and stir in the chocolate chips with a spoon.

Place the dough in the refrigerator to harden for about 30 minutes.

You have a few different options for serving:

Roll out the dough and use a cookie cutter to make fun shapes.

Shape the dough into balls and roll them in shredded coconut.

Or just serve it and enjoy!

Refrigerator Chocolate Macaroons

½ cup raw almonds or almond flour

1½ cups dried unsweetened coconut flakes, plus more for rolling
  if desired

½ cup cacao powder

½ cup raw organic honey, coconut nectar, or maple syrup

¼ cup coconut butter (this is the coconut meat blended with the
  oil, not just coconut oil)

1 teaspoon vanilla powder

Pinch of sea salt

Process the raw almonds in a food processor until they are finely chopped.
(If you are using the almond flour, omit this step.)

To the ground almonds, or flour, add the coconut flakes, cacao, honey,
coconut butter, vanilla powder, and salt. Process the mixture until it is
well blended but still has plenty of texture.

Using a mini ice cream scoop or a tablespoon, shape the mixture into
balls. At this point you may choose to roll them in extra shredded coconut.

Place the macaroons in the refrigerator to set, or alternatively dehydrate
them for about 8 to 10 hours in a dehydrator set to 115°F.

Fruit and Nut Super Chocolate Cups

½ cup cacao powder

¼ cup almond butter

1 tablespoon lucuma powder

¼ cup coconut oil, melted

2 tablespoons raw organic honey or your favorite sweetener

Handful of goji berries, goldenberries, raisins, nuts (cashews, macadamia nuts, almonds, pistachios, etc.), and/or hemp seeds, plus extra to use as garnishes

In a blender or food processor, process the cacao, almond butter, lucuma powder, coconut oil, and sweetener until the mixture is well combined. Transfer the mixture to a bowl, and stir in with a spoon or spatula your preferred assortment of dried fruits and nuts.

Fill mini baking cups with a spoonful of the chocolate mixture, and top each cup with a nut, some dried fruit, or a sprinkle of hemp seeds.

Place the cups in the refrigerator or freezer to set. These cups will store well if they are kept cold.

Easy No-Bake Brownies

These brownies are made from whole foods and contain no gluten, dairy, flour, or processed sugar.

- **1 pound raw almonds**
- **1 pound dates, pitted**
- **1 cup cacao powder or carob powder (or use half cacao and half carob)**
- **2 teaspoons vanilla powder**
- **1 teaspoon good-quality sea salt**
- **Up to 1 tablespoon superfood powder of your choice (optional)**
- **½ to 1 cup chopped nuts (almonds, hazelnuts, jungle peanuts, pecans, pine nuts, walnuts, etc.) and/or cacao nibs (optional)**
- **Coconut oil, for greasing**

In a food processor, combine the raw almonds, dates, cacao and/or carob powder, vanilla powder, salt, and superfood powder (if using). The dough should be smooth and slightly sticky.

Transfer the dough to a bowl, and stir in your choice of nuts and/or cacao nibs by hand.

Press the dough evenly into an 8 × 8-inch baking dish greased with coconut oil. You may want to have a little coconut oil on your fingers to keep the dough from sticking to your hands.

The dough can be scored for brownies and eaten right away or refrigerated to set and then cut into bars to enjoy. The brownies store well for a few weeks in the refrigerator or longer in the freezer.

Chocolate-Covered Strawberries

½ cup finely chopped cacao paste

1 tablespoon coconut oil, melted

Sweetener to taste (honey, maple syrup, etc.)

Pinch of good-quality sea salt

1 pound fresh strawberries or your favorite fruit, cleaned and dried thoroughly

Line a baking sheet with parchment paper and set aside.

In a double boiler or a saucepan set over low heat, melt the cacao paste. Transfer the melted paste to a bowl and quickly mix in the melted coconut oil, sweetener, and salt. Adjust sweetness as desired.

Dip the strawberries (or other fruit) in the melted cacao mix, leaving the top of each strawberry and its stem bare. Place each dipped strawberry on the lined baking sheet. Allow the strawberries to cool completely and harden at room temperature for a few hours, then refrigerate. Enjoy!

Raw Chocolate Pudding

1 large or 2 small ripe avocados, peeled and pitted

½ cup cacao powder or carob powder

⅓ cup coconut oil, melted

¼ cup coconut water

4 tablespoons raw organic honey

2 tablespoons xylitol or sun-dried cane juice crystals

½ teaspoon vanilla powder

Pinch of sea salt

Blend all the ingredients together in a high-speed blender until the mixture is smooth. Thin the pudding by adding more coconut water if desired. *The more oil and the less water used, the more fudgy the final product.*

Store the pudding in the refrigerator in an airtight container for up to a week, if you can keep it that long!

Easy Mocha Lovers' Tart

For the crust

> 1½ cups almond meal
> ¼ cup cacao powder
> ¼ cup coconut oil, melted
> 2 tablespoons raw organic honey
> 2 tablespoons maca powder
> 1 to 2 tablespoons ground chia seeds
> Pinch of sea salt

For the filling

> 2 medium avocados, peeled and pitted
> ½ cup cacao powder
> ⅓ cup coconut oil, melted
> ¼ cup strong coffee or coconut water
> 3 to 4 tablespoons raw organic honey
> 2 tablespoons coconut sugar
> Pinch of sea salt

To make the crust, process in a food processor all the crust ingredients until the dough is well combined and starts to stick together. Add a teaspoon of water if necessary to make it stick better. If you don't have a food processor, mix the ingredients by hand in a bowl, but make sure everything clumps together well before filling the tart pan.

Press the crust dough into a 9-inch tart pan, then place the tin in the refrigerator to set while you prepare the filling.

Blend together all the filling ingredients in a high-speed blender until the mixture is smooth. You can adjust the thickness and intensity of flavor by adding more or less coffee or coconut water. Adjust also for your preferred sweetness.

When the crust is ready, spoon in the filling mixture, spreading it evenly. You might opt to garnish the tart at this point with cacao nibs, chocolate chips, shredded coconut, or fresh berries.

Chill to set the tart. It will keep well, covered, in the refrigerator for up to a week.

Note: When the tart is stored in the fridge, it thickens due to the coconut oil. Plan for this accordingly by adjusting the ratio of liquid to oil you use in the recipe, depending on your desired density.

ACKNOWLEDGMENTS

Thank you so much to my extraordinary team for all your contributions and research that made this book possible:

R. A. Gauthier

Lucien Gauthier

Katherine Mottram

Krystyna Robin McMillan

A big thanks also to:

Ioana Aboumitri

Steve Adler

Angela Andrews

Anita Arze

Rebecca Astara

Barbara Barcelo

Jennifer Bartell

Etti Ben-Zion

Gina Berardino

Sasha Boussina

Gabrielle Brick

Justin Bua

Colleen Cackowski

Laura Capina

Adam Collins

Groovinda Dasi

Elynn DeMattia

Novak and Jelena Djokovic

Jason Doig

Solla Eiriks

Len Foley

Ronny Freedom

LaGita Groth

Elías Guðmundsson

Lars Gustafsson

Marcelo Hamui

Angela Hartman

Sarah Haugen

Jesse Herman

Sitara Hewitt

Rowena Jayne

Jack Jeffries

Simon and Maria Kirke

Debbie and Athena Kleven

Steff Lazar

Linda Lippi

Perla and Robert Machaen

Spencer Mack

Kimber Mahon
Doug Marshall
Andrea McGinnis
Soma Mission
Dena Hayes Mucha
Scott and Christi Mueller
Kai Nygard
Mia Peled
Solvi Petursson
Jonathon Porter
Emily Rakhit
Kevin Reyes

Dream Rockwell
Carolyn Solton
Gary Spirer
Karina Velasc
Franco Vescovi
Erin Waage
Tarran Webster
Christoffer Weiss
Jorgen Welsink
Ahava Wills
Crystal Wolfe
Mehrnoush Zolghadr

Thank you to my fellow health visionaries:

Daniel Aaron
Nadine Artemis
Gillian Brown
Kristina Carrilo-Bucaram
Kerrie Cushing
Chervin Jafarieh
Dr. Sara Gottfried
Russell Feingold
Brooke Hampton

Woody and Laura Harrelson
Andrea McNinch
Kimchi Moyler
Steve Sanna
Nicholas Tancheff
Ron Teeguarden
Robert Williams
Howard Wills
Jason Wrobel

A big shout-out to the amazing team at HarperOne:

Laina Adler
Yvonne Chan
Kim Dayman
Terri Leonard

Melinda Mullin
Suzanne Quist
Sydney Rogers
Gideon Weil

GLOSSARY

Acidic: The pH (potential hydrogen) scale ranges from 0.0 to 14.0, with 7.0 considered neutral. Anything with a pH between 0.0 and 7.0 is acidic. A variety of health issues arise from having an acidic system, such as a weakened immune system, chronic infection, heart disease, and digestive disorders. Also, bones will leach calcium in order to stabilize pH levels in the body, causing weakened bone strength and density as the body ages. The human digestive system is naturally acidic in order to break down food and extract nutrients, but ingesting processed and sugar-filled foods raises acidity in the body. A plant-based diet, free from processed foods, naturally balances the body's pH.

Adaptogen: This is a type of herb or food that gives the body a greater ability to adapt to stress or change and helps the body to maintain homeostasis. Most adaptogens grow in challenging environments that force the plant to develop adaptogenic phytochemicals to survive. Eating adaptogens is a crucial component of a beauty and longevity diet.

Alkaline: An alkaline system has a pH (potential hydrogen) over 7.0. The pH scale ranges from 0.0 to 14.0, with 7.0 considered a neutral pH, and a balanced system falls in the range between 7.0 and 7.4. Foods and spring water high in minerals are more alkaline. Since processed foods cause more acidity in the body, working toward a more mineralized alkaline diet is advisable. Eating a plant-based diet, free from processed foods, will naturally bring the body into pH balance.

Anthocyanin: This is the red, blue, or purple pigment found in many foods, such as berries. Foods with anthocyanins are natural antioxidants with neuroprotective power, benefitting the nervous system and eyesight.

Ayurveda: This profound system of health originated in India more than five thousand years ago. Ayurveda focuses on balancing the humors, or doshas, of the body through diet and lifestyle to produce radiant health and longevity. Every person possesses all the three doshas—kapha, pitta, and vata—but each in different strengths, making Ayurveda a highly personalized system of diet. In Ayurveda, disease can only arise from imbalances in the doshas. Through herbs, essential oils, activity levels, and foods, a person is easily able to balance their dominant dosha and allow harmony of the bodily elements to maintain health and freedom from disease.

Blood–brain barrier: This is the protective membrane that separates blood and other fluids from the brain. Select molecules are allowed to pass through the membrane, such as lipids and sugars that are essential for brain function, while toxins are kept out. Essential oils can penetrate this gatekeeper of the brain and can be used effectively in alternative health protocols.

BPA: Bisphenol A is a compound used in plastics. It is considered a hormone disruptor and a cause of increased estrogen levels and estrogen dominance. Since it mimics the hormone estrogen, it is aptly named a xenoestrogen. Although most food and personal care product companies are moving away from its use, the substitutes available are often as bad or worse than BPA, so research carefully before using so-called BPA-free products.

Cortisol: The adrenal glands produce this vital hormone. It is released during fight-or-flight stress responses and when consuming foods. Cortisol plays a large role in energy production and fat storage, and a balanced cortisol level is necessary for optimal health. Elevated cortisol can reduce immune function, cause belly fat, and adversely affect mood.

Cytokine: This is a protein cell signaler that mobilizes the body's immune system response. In the course of a normal immune response, cytokines are essential; however, toxicity can cause fat cells to release cytokines, creating rampant inflammation.

EFAs: Essential fatty acids are so named because they are essential for biological function. They must be consumed through diet since the body cannot make EFAs on its own.

Enteric nervous system: Known as the "second brain," this part of the autonomic nervous system is imbedded in the walls of the gut and can act independently of the brain. It possesses intelligence and is linked to our emotions and our interpretation of the external, such as when we say we have a "gut feeling" about something.

Enzyme: An enzyme is a protein that facilitates chemical reactions in the body. There are two main types: metabolic and digestive. It is important to replenish the body's enzyme "bank account" with whole fresh fruits and vegetables. Raw foods are rich in enzymes, which is why they spoil so quickly. Foods low in enzymes, like processed foods, have a longer shelf life.

Flavonoid: These plant-based nutrients are found in virtually all fruits and vegetables. They are responsible for the health benefits associated with fruits and vegetables and are essential for a healthy diet.

Flavonol: This is a type of flavonoid that contains aromatic phytonutrients. One of the highest concentrations of flavonols can be found in raw cacao.

Glycation: This linking of a sugar molecule with a protein or fat leads to degradation of cellular structures. When glycation occurs in the skin, it produces a leathery texture. Protein or lipids that become glycated are called "advanced glycation end products" (AGEs). Glycation can be avoided by eating carbs and sugars in moderation as well as few or no foods cooked at high temperatures, meaning fried, grilled, or toasted.

GMO: A genetically modified organism is a plant that has been modified via manipulation of its genes. The most common GMO crops are soy, corn, rapeseed, wheat, and cotton. Many European and Asian countries have banned GMO products. In the US, GMOs are currently not subject to federal labeling laws, so care is needed when purchasing products containing the previously mentioned ingredients.

Hormone: The "master switches" of the body, hormones signal critical functions and regulate homeostasis. Commonly associated with growth and development, hormones also regulate metabolism and energy. Balancing the hormones is crucial since they act in concert with one another. Hormones are also a definitive marker for health; elevated or deficient hormone levels are sure to adversely affect both health and appearance.

Inflammation: Also known as "false fire" in Traditional Chinese Medicine, inflammation is the swelling of tissue in response to unnatural or harmful occurrences in the body. Pathogens, injury, and infection cause the body to produce an inflammatory response to eliminate the danger or repair cellular damage. Chronic inflammation is the most dangerous type of inflammation because, unchecked, inflammation over a long period of time will damage the body itself.

LDL cholesterol: Low-density lipoprotein is also widely known as the "bad" cholesterol. If LDL particles oxidize, they can clog and damage arteries, causing the progression of heart disease. Saturated fats were long demonized as raising LDL cholesterol, but this correlation is now regarded as unsubstantiated.

Linoleic acid: This is an omega-6 fatty acid that cannot be made by the body but must come from whole food sources. An example of this omega-6 is gamma-linoleic acid (GLA). They are found in seeds, nuts, and oils like pumpkin seed, walnuts, and pine nuts.

Linolenic acid: This omega-3 fatty acid, also known as alpha-linolenic acid (ALA), comes from plant-based sources. It can be derived from recommended sources, like hemp and chia, or from nonrecommended industrial oils, like soybean and canola, which are degraded and dangerous.

Lipid: Generally speaking, a lipid is a fat or fatty acid, though fats are a subgroup within lipids since lipids can also include fat-soluble vitamins and other compounds, such as waxes.

Lymph node: Also known as a lymph gland, this small sac regulates the flow of lymph fluid. The human body typically has more than five hundred lymph nodes. As lymph fluid moves through the body and the lymph nodes, waste and toxins are filtered out. Since the body has more lymph than blood, this filtration system is vital for the immune system and health.

Medicinal mushroom: A mushroom or fungal mycelium that grows primarily on trees and contains unique phytochemicals that "teach" the immune system, making it more intelligent. Reishi and chaga are considered the queen and king of the medicinal mushroom world. They cannot be eaten but must be decocted to extract the essential nutrients.

Melanocyte: A cell that produces melanin is a melanocyte. These cells are responsible for skin color and pigmentation.

Microbiome: This is the community of bacteria that resides inside the body, such as in the gut, as well as outside the body, such as on the surface of the skin. The health of the microbiome determines the over-all health and vitality of the entire body. If the microbiome is weak or unhealthy, ill health is imminent. Eating fresh, whole, and fermented foods replenishes beneficial bacteria in the body and can be supple-mented with probiotics.

ORAC scale: The oxygen radical absorbance capacity scale measures the antioxidant capacity of foods. The higher the score, the higher the ability of that food to fight free radicals. Foods with a high ORAC score are ideal to incorporate into your diet. These consist of berries, medic-inal mushrooms, superfoods, and superherbs.

Progesterone: This "beauty hormone" is also considered a primary sex hormone. It is found in both men and women, and is involved with mood and sex drive. Plus, it plays a pivotal role in pregnancy for women. Progesterone balances estrogen and must be kept at a normal level to avoid estrogen dominance.

Squalene: This is an oil concentrated in the nervous system and brain. Found in olive oil, squalene is an antioxidant and a beauty enhancer.

Telomere: This is an endcap on a chromosome that protects that chromosome against DNA damage and facilitates cellular replication. As we age, telomeres get shorter and shorter. A healthy diet and low stress help to slow down the shortening process. Telomeres are at the forefront of longevity and anti-aging research.

Testosterone: This is the primary sex hormone for men; it controls sex drive, mood, energy, and motivation. As testosterone diminishes over time, a decrease in all these occurs and andropause develops unless appropriate action is taken.

Xenoestrogen: These are chemicals that mimic the hormone estrogen and disrupt the normal functions of our body. Typically they cause unwanted growths and send false signals to the body. They are also a type of "endocrine disruptor." Examples of xenoestrogens are BPA, PCBs, and phthalates, and are most commonly found in plastics.

RESOURCES

Longevity Warehouse

http://www.longevitywarehouse.com

Longevity Warehouse® is an online wellness superstore offering the highest-integrity organic and wild-crafted foods from the cleanest sources available on earth. Our mission is to provide access to the best-quality superfoods, superherbs, and other natural lifestyle prod-ucts, at the lowest possible prices, so you can take your health to the next level. We also strive to educate through cutting-edge articles, recipes, and blog posts to help you make informed decisions about your health and add more years to your life and more life to your years.

The Longevity Now® Conference

http://www.thelongevitynowconference.com

The Longevity Now® Conference is the premier wellness event in the world, featuring experts in the fields of anti-aging, rejuvenation, and longevity. Held once a year, this event offers the most innovative longevity ideas, tools, and technologies by featuring world-renowned health and wellness experts and by gathering in our exhibitor hall high-integrity companies whose products contribute to the superior well-being of others, enhance peak performance, and are eco-friendly and sustainable. Also featured is our state-of-the-art Longevity Tonic Bar™ where elixir masterminds share their most coveted secret concoctions for creating refreshing tonics, herbal coffees, and nourishing elixirs using powerful superfoods and superherbs that provide premium nutrition on a cellular level.

Women's Wellness Conference™

http://www.womenswellnessconference.com
The Women's Wellness Conference™ is the leading women's health event in the United States, featuring experts and visionaries who explore numerous critical women's mind and body topics, such as vibrant health, metabolic function, anti-aging, nutrition, beauty, digestion, adrenal health, detoxification, the microbiome, relationships, epigenetics, fitness, immune-system health, and more! Exploring new themes each event, participants learn how to comprehensively upgrade their wellness program, no matter where they are in their personal journey. The conference also features the famous Longevity Tonic Bar™ and endorses a select group of conscious exhibitors whose products contribute to optimum health and well-being and are sustainable and organic or wild-crafted.

The Fruit Tree Planting Foundation

www.ftpf.org
The Fruit Tree Planting Foundation is a nonprofit charity dedicated to planting edible, fruitful trees and plants to benefit needy populations and improve the surrounding air, soil, and water.

David Wolfe's Raw Nutrition Certification Course

https://bodymindinstitute.com/the-exclusive-david-wolfe-nutrition -certification

Other Books by David Wolfe

Eating for Beauty, The Sunfood Diet Success System, Superfoods: The Food and Medicine of the Future, Naked Chocolate, Chaga: King of the Medicinal Mushrooms, and *Longevity Now.*

Documentaries Featuring David Wolfe

Food Matters, Hungry for Change, Discover the Gift, The Frequency of Genius, The Raw Natural, Simply Raw: Reversing Diabetes in 30 Days, Serpent and the Sun, Semisweet: Life in Chocolate, and *GMOs Revealed.*

Helpful Websites

The Beauty Diet book website: **www.beautydietbook.com**

Earthing™ information and products: **https://www.longevity warehouse.com/earthing**

Environmental Working Group: **https://www.ewg.org**

EWG's Skin Deep Cosmetics Database: **https://www.ewg.org/skindeep**

Hormone testing: **https://www.canaryclub.org**

REFERENCES

The following references are listed in the order used within the book.

Introduction: The Five Beauty Factors

Sorvino, Chloe. "Why the $445 Billion Beauty Industry Is a Gold Mine for Self-Made Women." *Forbes*, May 18, 2017. Accessed November 13, 2017. https://www.forbes.com/sites/chloesorvino/2017/05/18/self-made-women-wealth-beauty-gold-mine/#348601d72a3a.

Environmental Working Group. "Personal Care Products Safety Act Would Improve Cosmetics Safety." Accessed July 20, 2017. http://www.ewg.org/Personal-Care-Products-Safety-Act-Would-Improve-Cosmetics-Safety#.WdLz6miPKUk.

Beauty Factor 1: Eat for Beauty

Erb, Kelly Phillips. "More Americans Believe It's Easier to Understand Tax than How to Eat Healthy." *Forbes*, May 23, 2012. Accessed October 31, 2017. https://www.forbes.com/sites/kellyphillipserb/2012/05/23/more-americans-believe-its-easier-to-understand-tax-than-how-to-eat-healthy/#5977a6316d12.

Matthews, Jania. "Americans Find Doing Their Own Taxes Simpler than Improving Diet and Health." International Food Information Council Foundation, May 22, 2012. Last modified May 23, 2014. http://www.foodinsight.org/Americans_Find_Doing_Their_Own_Taxes_Simpler_Than_Improving_Diet_and_Health.

Blodget, Henry. "Chart of the Day: American Per-Capita Sugar Consumption Hits 100 Pounds per Year." Business Insider, February 19, 2012. Accessed July 17, 2017. http://www.businessinsider.com/chart-american-sugar-consumption-2012-2#IXZZ1X9SZDPKK.

KGB Answers. "How Many Skittles Make a Pound." January 19, 2017. Accessed July 17, 2017. http://www.kgbanswers.com/how-many-skittles-make-a-pound/7532970.

Cespedes, Andrea. "How Many Calories Are in One Gram of Sugar?" Livestrong.com, September 27, 2013. Accessed July 17, 2017. http://www.livestrong.com/article /292069-calories-in-a-pack-of-sugar/.

Associated Press. "Cut Back, Way Back, on Sugar, Says Heart Group." NBC News, August 24, 2009. Accessed July 17, 2017. http://www.msnbc.msn.com/id /32543288/ns/health-diet_and_nutrition/t/cut-back-way-back-sugar-says -health-group?#.t9e7uplyvqw.

Anne, Melodie. "How Many Teaspoons of Sugar Are There in a Can of Coke?" Livestrong.com, April 14, 2015. Accessed July 17, 2017. http://www.livestrong .com/article/283136-how-many-teaspoons-of-sugar-are-there-in-a-can-of-coke/.

Sugar Stacks. "Would You Eat a Stack of 16 Sugar Cubes?" 2009. Accessed July 17, 2017. http://www.sugarstacks.com.

Herr, Norman. "Television and Health." California State University, Northridge, 2007. Accessed July 17, 2017. http://www.csun.edu/science/health/docs/tv &health.html.

Goldwert, Lindsay. "Sugar Is as Addictive as Cocaine, and Causes Obesity, Diabetes, Cancer, and Heart Disease: Researchers." *NY Daily News*, April 2, 2012. Accessed July 17, 2017. http://www.nydailynews.com/life-style/health/researcher-sugar -addictive-cocaine-obesity-diabetes-cancer-heart-disease-article-1.1054419.

Taubes, Gary. "Is Sugar Toxic?" *New York Times*, April 13, 2011. Accessed July 20, 2017. http://www.nytimes.com/2011/04/17/magazine/mag-17Sugar-t.html.

Consumer Reports. "Health Risks of Protein Drinks." Last modified July 2010. https:// www.consumerreports.org/cro/2012/04/protein-drinks/index.htm.

Kristo, A. A., D. Klimis-Zacas, and A. K. Sikalidis. "Protective Role of Dietary Berries in Cancer." *Antioxidants* (Basel) 5, no. 4 (2016): 37.

Mercola, Joseph. "What Are Sprouts Good For?" Food Facts. Accessed July 20, 2017. http://foodfacts.mercola.com/sprouts.html.

Cousens, Gabriel. *Conscious Eating*. 2nd ed. Berkeley: North Atlantic Books, 2000.

Heinerman, John. *Heinerman's Encyclopedia of Healing Juices*. Paramus, NJ: Reward Books, 1994.

Onstad, Dianne. *Whole Foods Companion*. White River Junction, VT: Chelsea Green, 1996.

Shazzie. *Detox Your World.* 2nd ed. Norwich, UK: Rawcreation, 2003.

Bjarnadottir, Adda. "5 Studies on Saturated Fat—Time to Retire the Myth?" Health-line, August 18, 2016. Accessed July 29, 2017. http://www.healthline.com /nutrition/5-studies-on-saturated-fat#section1.

Superfoods and Superherbs: The Building Blocks of Beauty

De Rosso, V. V., S. Hillebrand, E. Cuevas Montilla, F. O. Bobbio, P. Winterhalter, and A. Z. Mercadante. "Determination of Anthocyanins from Acerola (*Malpighia Emarginata DC.*) and Acai (*Euterpe Oleracea Mart.*) by HPLC-PDA-MS/MS." *Journal of Food Composition and Analysis* 21, no. 4 (2008): 291–99.

De Souza, M. O., L. Souza e Silva, C. L. de Brito Magalhães, B. B. de Figueiredo, D. C. Costa, M. E. Silva, and M. L. Pedrosa. "The Hypocholesterolemic Activity of Acai (*Euterpe Oleracea Mart.*) Is Mediated by the Enhanced Expression of the ATP-Binding Cassette, Subfamily G Transporters 5 and 8, and Low-Density Lipopro-tein Receptor Genes in the Rat." *Nutrition Research* 32, no. 12 (2012): 976–84.

Foster, Meika, Duncan Hunter, and Samir Samman. "Evaluation of the Nutritional and Metabolic Effects of Aloe Vera." In *Herbal Medicine: Biomolecular and Clinical Aspects*, 2nd ed., edited by Iris F. F. Benzie and Sissi Wachtel-Galor, Boca Raton, FL: CRC Press/Taylor and Francis, 2011. https://www.ncbi.nlm.nih.gov/books /NBK92765/#ch3_r81.

Byeon, S. W., R. P. Pelley, S. E. Ullrich, T. A. Waller, C. D. Bucana, and F. M. Strick-land. "*Aloe Barbadensis* Extracts Reduce the Production of Interleukin-10 After Exposure to Ultraviolet Radiation." *Journal of Investigative Dermatology* 110, no. 5 (1998): 811–17.

Feily, A., and M. R. Namazi. "Aloe Vera in Dermatology: A Brief Review." *Giornale Italiano di Dermatologia e Venereologia* 144, no. 1 (2009): 85–91.

University of California Agriculture and Natural Resources. "Avocado Information: General Information." Accessed July 28, 2017. http://ucavo.ucr.edu/general /historyname.html.

Sturluson, Thordur. "Avocado Medicinal Use and Benefits." Herbal Resource. Accessed July 29, 2017. https://www.herbal-supplement-resource.com/avocado -medicinal-uses.html.

CureJoy Editorial. "9 Surprising Benefits of Avocado Seeds You Should Tap Into."

CureJoy, June 7, 2017. Accessed July 29, 2017. https://www.curejoy.com/content/avocado-seed-benefits/.

Sexton, Shannon. "Your Guide to Ayurvedic Massage Oils." Yoga International, May 9, 2013. Accessed July 29, 2017. https://yogainternational.com/article/view/your-guide-to-ayurvedic-massage-oils.

Ware, Megan. "12 Health Benefits of Avocado." Medical News Today. Reviewed by Natalie Olsen. Last modified September 12, 2017. https://www.medicalnewstoday.com/articles/270406.php.

Dreher, M. L., and A. J. Davenport. "Hass Avocado Composition and Potential Health Effects." *Critical Reviews in Food Science and Nutrition* 53, no. 7 (2013): 738–50.

M., Renu. "17 Amazing Benefits of Cacao for Skin, Hair, and Health." StyleCraze, September 20, 2017. Accessed July 22, 2017. http://www.stylecraze.com/articles/amazing-benefits-of-cacao-for-skin-hair-and-health/#gref.

Skae, Teya. "Examining the Properties of Chocolate and Cacao for Health." Natural News, February 7, 2008. Accessed July 22, 2017. https://www.naturalnews.com/022610_cacao_chocolate_raw.html.

St. Jean, Julie. "Medicinal and Ritualistic Uses for Chocolate in Mesoamerica." HeritageDaily. Accessed July 22, 2017. http://www.heritagedaily.com/2015/08/medicinal-and-ritualistic-uses-for-chocolate-in-mesoamerica-2/98809.

Alban, Deane. "Anandamide: Putting the Bliss Molecule to Work for Your Brain." Reset.me, March 29, 2016. Accessed July 22, 2017. http://reset.me/story/anandamide-putting-the-bliss-molecule-to-work-for-your-brain/.

Raloff, Janet. "Chocolate as Sunscreen." *Food for Thought* (blog). *Science News*, June 7, 2006. Accessed October 10, 2017. https://www.sciencenews.org/blog/food-thought/chocolate-sunscreen.

Vince, Gaia. "Eating Chocolate May Halve Risk of Dying," *New Scientist*, February 27, 2006. http://www.newscientist.com/channel/health/dn8780.html. (Citing B. Buijsse, E. J. M. Feskens, F. J. Kok, and D. Kromhout. "Cocoa Intake, Blood Pressure, and Cardiovascular Mortality: The Zutphen Elderly Study." *Archives of Internal Medicine* 166, no. 4 (2006): 411–17.)

Erasmus, Udo. *Fats That Heal, Fats That Kill.* Burnaby, British Columbia: Alive Books, 2001.

PopSugar. "21 Unexpected Beauty Uses for Coconut Oil." *Allure*, April 11, 2014.

Accessed July 27, 2017. https://www.allure.com/story/beauty-uses-for -coconut-oil.

Rekstis, Emily. "I Tried 9 Coconut Oil Beauty Hacks for a Week So You Don't Have To." *Self*, February 19, 2016. Accessed July 27, 2017. http://www.self.com/story /coconut-oil-beauty-hacks.

Keshav. "History of Coconut Oil." The Superfoods. Accessed July 27, 2017. https:// www.thesuperfoods.net/coconut/history-of-coconut-oil.

Wilcox, Christie. "Hawaiian Health and the Coconut." Nutrition Wonderland, July 7, 2009. Accessed July 27, 2017. http://nutritionwonderland.com/2009/07 /hawaiian-health-coconut/.

Niu, A. J., J. M. Wu, D. H. Yu, and R. Wang. "Protective Effect of *Lycium Barbarum* Polysaccharides on Oxidative Damage in Skeletal Muscle of Exhaustive Exercise Rats." *International Journal of Biological Macromolecules* 42, no. 5 (2008): 447–49.

Mindell, Earl, and Rick Handel. *Goji: The Himalayan Health Secret*. Lake Dallas, TX: Momentum Media, 2003. Accessed July 20, 2017, via Goji Health Singapore. http://www.gojihealthsingapore.com/Research-Supported%20Uses%20of%20 Goji.pdf.

Yin, G., and Y. Dang. "Optimization of Extraction Technology of the *Lycium Barbarum* Polysaccharides by Box–Behnken Statistical Design." *Carbohydrate Polymers* 74, no. 3 (2008): 603–10.

Jiao, R., Y. Liu, H. Gao, J. Xiao, and K. F. So. "The Antioxidant and Antitumor Properties of Plant Polysaccharides." *American Journal of Chinese Medicine* 44, no. 3 (2016): 463–88.

Erasmus. *Fats That Heal*.

Suzar (Dr. S. Epps). *Drugs Masquerading as Foods*. Ojai, CA: A-Kar Productions, 1999.

Zavasta, Tonya. "Raw Hemp Hearts, aka Shelled Hemp Seeds: A 'Super-Food' with Real Health Benefits." Beautiful on Raw. Accessed July 23, 2017. http://www .beautifulonraw.com/hemp-seeds.html.

Z Living Staff. "9 Health Benefits of Hemp Oil That You Should Know." Z Living, June 3, 2015. Accessed July 23, 2017. http://www.zliving.com/wellness/natural -remedies/9-health-benefits-of-hemp-oil-that-you-should-know.

University of Maryland Medical Center. "Gamma-Linolenic Acid." Medical Reference Guide. Last modified June 22, 2015. Accessed October 10, 2017. http://www.umm .edu/health/medical/altmed/supplement/gammalinolenic-acid.

Cooper, R. A., P. C. Molan, and K. G. Harding. "The Sensitivity to Honey of Gram-Positive Cocci of Clinical Significance Isolated from Wounds." *Journal of Applied Microbiology* 93, no. 5 (2002): 857–63.

Cooper, R. A., E. Halas, and P. C. Molan. "The Efficacy of Honey in Inhibiting Strains of *Pseudomonas Aeruginosa* from Infected Burns." *Journal of Burn Care Rehabilitation* 23, no. 6 (2002): 366–70.

Ahmed, A. K., M. J. Hoekstra, J. J. Hage, and R. B. Karim. "Honey-Medicated Dressing: Transformation of an Ancient Remedy into Modern Therapy." *Annals of Plastic Surgery* 50, no. 2 (2003): 143–47, discussion 147–48.

Natarajan, S., D. Williamson, J. Grey, K. G. Harding, and R. A. Cooper. "Healing of an MRSA-Colonized, Hydroxyurea-Induced Leg Ulcer with Honey." *Journal of Dermatological Treatment* 12, no. 1 (2001): 33–36.

Dunford, C., R. Cooper, and P. Molan. "Using Honey as a Dressing for Infected Skin Lesions." *Nursing Times* 96, suppl. 14 (2000): 7–9.

Traynor, Joe. *Honey, The Gourmet Medicine.* Bakersfield, CA: Kovak Books, 2002.

Loux, Renee. "11 Ways to Use Honey to Get More Gorgeous Skin, Hair, and Nails." *Women's Health*, September 25, 2014. Accessed July 26, 2017. http://www.womenshealthmag.com/beauty/beauty-uses-for-honey.

Padykula, Jessica. "No DIY Disasters Here—The Beauty Benefits of Honey Are Real." SheKnows. Last modified October 23, 2017. Accessed July 26, 2017. http://www.sheknows.com/beauty-and-style/articles/1017621/beauty-benefits-of-honey.

Williams, Colleen. "16 Ways to Use Honey as a Beauty Product." YouBeauty, December 1, 2014. Accessed July 26, 2017. http://www.youbeauty.com/beauty/16-ways-you-never-thought-to-use-honey-as-a-beauty-product/.

Mandal, M. D., and S. Mandal. "Honey: Its Medicinal Property and Antibacterial Activity." *Asian Pacific Journal of Tropical Biomedicine* 1, no. 2 (2011): 154–60.

Eteraf-Oskouei, T., and M. Najafi. "Traditional and Modern Uses of Natural Honey in Human Diseases: A Review." *Iranian Journal of Basic Medical Sciences* 16, no. 6 (2013): 731–42.

Palmer, Alice. "Honey: The Facts." *Runner's World*, May 7, 2010. Accessed July 26, 2017. https://www.runnersworld.co.uk/nutrition/honey-the-facts.

Ley, Beth M. Maca: *Adaptogen and Hormonal Regulator*. Minneapolis: BL Publications, 2003.

Lapidos, Rachel. "The One Superherb to Try for a Seriously Big Beauty Boost." Well+Good, April 11, 2017. Accessed July 24, 2017. https://www.wellandgood .com/good-looks/maca-skin-hair-beauty-benefits/.

Palsdottir, Hrefna. "9 Benefits of Maca Root (and Potential Side Effects)." Healthline, October 30, 2016. Accessed July 24, 2017. https://www.healthline.com/nutrition /benefits-of-maca-root#section1.

Rodriguez, Hethir. "Maca, Wonder Herb for Fertility." Natural Fertility Info, June 2016. Accessed October 10, 2017. http://natural-fertility-info.com/maca.

Zhang, Diana, and Diane Zhang. "10 Ancient Uses of Olive Oil." *Epoch Times*. Last modified November 8, 2013. Accessed July 21, 2017. http://www.theepochtimes .com/n3/228883–10-ancient-uses-of-olive-oil/.

Lewis, Linnea. "The Many Uses of Olive Oil in Ancient Rome." HubPages, December 10, 2015. Accessed July 21, 2017. https://hubpages.com/education/The-Many -Uses-of-Olive-Oil-in-Ancient-Rome.

Explore Crete. "History of Olive Oil." Accessed July 21, 2017. http://www.explorecrete .com/nature/olive-oil-history.html.

International Olive Council. "Olive Oil and Cardiovascular Diseases." Accessed July 21, 2017. http://www.internationaloliveoil.org/estaticos/view/88-olive-oil -and-cardiovascular-diseases.

Heinerman, John. *Dr. Heinerman's Encyclopedia of Nature's Vitamins and Minerals*. Paramus, NJ: Prentice Hall, 1998.

Axford, S., O. Mutton, and A. Adams. "Beyond Pumpkin Seeds." *British Journal of Psychiatry* 158, no. 4 (1991): 573.

Brusie, Chaunie. "The Health Benefits of Pumpkin Seed Oil." Healthline, June 10, 2016. Accessed July 30, 2017. https://www.healthline.com/health/pumpkin -seed-oil.

Cho, Y. H., S. Y. Lee, D. W. Jeong, E. J. Choi, Y. J. Kim, J. G. Lee, Y. H. Yi, and H. S. Cha. "Effect of Pumpkin Seed Oil on Hair Growth in Men with Androgenetic Alopecia: A Randomized, Double-Blind, Placebo-Controlled Trial." *Evidence-Based Complementary and Alternative Medicine* (2014): 549721. Accessed July 30, 2017. https:// www.ncbi.nlm.nih.gov/pmc/articles/PMC4017725/.

Bachstetter, A. D., J. Jemberg, A. Schlunk, J. L. Vila, C. Hudson, M. J. Cole, R. D. Shytle, et al. "Spirulina Promotes Stem Cell Genesis and Protects Against LPS Induced Declines in Neural Stem Cell Proliferation." *PLOS One* 5, no. 5 (2010): e10496.

UC Davis Health. "UC Davis Study Shows Spirulina Boosts Immune System." News release. December 1, 2000. Accessed October 10, 2017. https://www.ucdmc .ucdavis.edu/publish/news/newsroom/2658.

Cheng-Wu, Z., T. Chao-Tsi, and Z. Zhen. "The Effects of Polysaccharide and Phyco-cyanin from Spirulina *Platensis* on Peripheral Blood and Hematopoietic System of Bone Marrow in Mice." *Proceedings of the Second Asia-Pacific Conference on Algal Biotechnology.* National University of Singapore, April 25–27, 1994, p. 58.

Leech, Joe. "10 Health Benefits of Spirulina." Healthline, June 4, 2017. Accessed July 25, 2017. https://www.healthline.com/nutrition/10-proven-benefits-of-spirulina.

US Department of Agriculture. "Basic Report: 11667, Seaweed, Spirulina, Dried." National Nutrient Database for Standard Reference Release 28. Accessed October 31, 2017. https://ndb.nal.usda.gov/ndb/foods/show/3306?fgcd=&manu =&lfacet=&format=&count=&max=50&offset=&sort=default&order=asc &qlookup=11667&ds=&qt=&qp=&qa=&qn=&q=&ing=.

US Department of Agriculture. "Basic Report: 23568, Beef, Ground, 85% Lean Meat/15% Fat, Patty, Cooked, Broiled." National Nutrient Database for Standard Reference Release 28. Accessed October 31, 2017. https://ndb.nal.usda.gov/ndb /foods/show/7612?fgcd=&manu=&lfacet=&format=&count=&max=50&offset =&sort=default&order=asc&qlookup=23568&ds=&qt=&qp=&qa=&qn=&q =&ing=.

Walansky, Aly. "10 Reasons Spirulina Is Your Body's Awesome Secret Weapon." StyleCaster, 2014. Accessed July 25, 2017. http://stylecaster.com/beauty /spirulina/.

Niyogi, Sreejan Guha. "I Had 'Amla' for a Month and Here's What It Does It Your Hair and Skin." BollywoodShaadis.com. Last modified October 12, 2017. Accessed August 2, 2017. http://www.bollywoodshaadis.com/articles/beautiful-and -amazing-reasons-to-add-amla-to-your-grocery-list-right-now-3219.

Choudhary, Tanya. "31 Amazing Benefits of Amla Juice for Skin, Hair, and Health." StyleCraze, September 19, 2017. Accessed August 2, 2017. http://www.stylecraze .com/articles/benefits-of-amla-juice-for-skin-hair-and-health/#gref.

Bhatia, Vidhi. "History." *Amla for Life* (blog). Accessed August 2, 2017. http://amlaforlife.blogspot.com/p/history.html.

Reddy, Catherine. "All About Amla (*Emblica Officinalis*)." *Earth of India,* September 21, 2012. Accessed August 2, 2017. http://theindianvegan.blogspot.com/2012/09/all-about-amla.html.

Chandrasekhar, K., J. Kapoor, and S. Anishetty. "A Prospective, Randomized Double-Blind, Placebo-Controlled Study of Safety and Efficacy of a High-Concentration Full-Spectrum Extract of Ashwagandha Root in Reducing Stress and Anxiety in Adults." *Indian Journal of Psychological Medicine* 34, no. 3 (2012): 255–62.

Bhattacharya, S. K., A. Bhattacharya, K. Sairam, and S. Ghosal. "Anxiolytic-Antidepressant Activity of *Withania Somnifera* Glycowithanolides: An Experimental Study." *Phytomedicine: International Journal of Phytotherapy and Phytopharmacology* 7, no. 6 (2000): 463–69.

Schelling, Christianne. "Herbal Help for Beautiful Skin." Ashwagandha.com. Accessed August 4, 2017. https://www.ashwagandha.com/natural-beauty/192-herbal-help-for-beautiful-skin.

Deshmukh, Chandrama. "36 Amazing Benefits of Ashwagandha for Skin, Hair, and Health." StyleCraze. Last modified November 13, 2017. http://www.stylecraze.com/articles/amazing-benefits-of-ashwagandha-for-skin-hair-and-health/#gref.

Ahuja, Aashna. "Ashwagandha: It's Powerful Health and Beauty Benefits You Didn't Know About." NDTV. Last modified October 15, 2017. http://food.ndtv.com/ayurveda/ashwagandha-the-powerful-health-benefits-and-beauty-benefits-you-need-to-know-1220328.

Schafer, Peg. *The Chinese Medicinal Herb Farm.* White River Junction, VT: Chelsea Green, 2011.

Teeguarden, Ron. *The Ancient Wisdom of the Chinese Tonic Herbs.* New York: Warner Books, 1998.

Ahmed, Arshi. "Top 10 Amazing Health Benefits of Longan." StyleCraze. Last modified September 19, 2017. http://www.stylecraze.com/articles/top-10-amazing-health-benefits-of-longan/#gref.

Teeguarden. *The Ancient Wisdom of the Chinese Tonic Herbs.*

Tierra, Michael. "Dragon's Eyes—Longan Berries." East West School of Planetary

Herbology. Accessed August 7, 2017. http://www.planetherbs.com/michaels -blog/dragons-eyes-longan-berries.html.

CureJoy Editorial. "6 Health Benefits and Uses of Neem Oil for Skin, Hair, and Health." CureJoy. Last modified September 1, 2017. https://www.curejoy.com /content/benefits-of-neem-oil-for-skin-hair-and-health/.

Neem Foundation. "History of Usage." Accessed August 1, 2017. http://www .neemfoundation.org/about-neem/history-of-usage/.

Franco, P., M. Rampino, O. Ostellino, M. Schena, G. Pecorari, P. Garzino Demo, M. Fasolis, et al. "Management of Acute Skin Toxicity with *Hypericum Perforatum* and Neem Oil During Platinum-Based Concurrent Chemo-Radiation in Head and Neck Cancer Patients." *Medical Oncology* 34, no. 2 (2017): 30.

Läuchli, S., S. Vannotti, J. Hafner, T. Hunziker, and L. French. "A Plant-Derived Wound Therapeutic for Cost-Effective Treatment of Post-Surgical Scalp Wounds with Exposed Bone." *Forschende Komplementärmedizin* 21, no. 2 (2014): 88–93.

The Indian Spot. "Herbal Remedies—Neem for Skin and Hair." Accessed August 1, 2017. https://theindianspot.com/herbal-remedies-neem-for-skin-and-hair/.

Artemis, Nadine. *Holistic Dental Care: The Complete Guide to Healthy Teeth and Gums.* Berkeley: North Atlantic Books, 2013.

Teeguarden. *The Ancient Wisdom of the Chinese Tonic Herbs.*

Jian-Ping, D., C. Jun, B. Yu-Fei, H. Bang-Xing, G. Shang-Bin, and J. Li-Li. "Effects of Pearl Powder Extract and Its Fractions on Fibroblast Function Relevant to Wound Repair." *Pharmaceutical Biology* 48, no. 2 (2010): 122–27.

Cohen, M. M. "Tulsi—*Ocimum Sanctum*: A Herb for All Reasons." *Journal of Ayurveda and Integrative Medicine* 5, no. 4 (2014): 251–59.

Tadimalla, Ravi Teja. "26 Amazing Benefits of Tulsi/Basil for Skin, Hair, and Health—A Must Use Herb." StyleCraze, September 28, 2017. Accessed August 3, 2017. http://www.stylecraze.com/articles/amazing-benefits-of-tulsibasil-for -skin-hair-and-health/#gref.

Saraswat, Kriti. "4 Ways Tulsi or Basil Can Help Enhance Your Beauty." TheHealth Site. Last modified November 18, 2015. Accessed August 3, 2017. http://www .thehealthsite.com/beauty/beauty-benefits-tulsi-basil-k114/.

Prakashan, Priya. "Beauty Benefits of Tulsi: 5 Ways Using Holy Basil Will Give You Healthy Skin and Hair." India.com, June 22, 2017. Accessed August 3, 2017.

http://www.india.com/lifestyle/beauty-benefits-of-tulsi-5-ways-using-holy
-basil-will-give-you-healthy-skin-and-hair-2260728/.

Nair, Aparna. "Tulsi Has Environmental Benefits Too." *The Times of India,* April 8,
2012. Accessed August 3, 2017. http://timesofindia.indiatimes.com/home
/environment/flora-fauna/Tulsi-has-environmental-benefits-too/articleshow
/12574905.cms.

Teeguarden. *The Ancient Wisdom of the Chinese Tonic Herbs.*

Smarty. "White Peony Root: The Anti-Aging Herb." Smart Living Network, December 4, 2007. Accessed August 6, 2017. https://www.smartlivingnetwork.com
/senior-health/b/white-peony-root-the-anti-aging-herb/.

Shen-Nong. "Chinese Herb List—*Radix Paeoniae Alba.*" Accessed August 6, 2017.
http://www.shen-nong.com/eng/herbal/baishaoyao.html.

Petter, Dawn. "Love Peonies? White Peony Root Is Being Used as Herbal Medicine."
Garden Collage Magazine, November 19, 2016. Accessed August 6, 2017. http://
gardencollage.com/heal/botanical-medicine/love-peonies-white-peony-root
-used-herbal-medicine/.

Beauty Factor 2: Remove Toxins

Collier, R. "Intermittent Fasting: The Science of Going Without." *Canadian Medical
Association Journal* 185, no. 9 (2013): E363–64.

Vighi, G., F. Marcucci, L. Sensi, G. Di Cara, and F. Frati. "Allergy and the Gastrointestinal System." *Clinical* and *Experimental Immunology* 153, suppl. 1 (2008): 3–6.

Hippocrates Health Institute. "Colon Hydrotherapy." Accessed November 20, 2017.
https://hippocratesinst.org/colon-hydrotherapy-2.

Tjandra, J. J., M. Chan, and P. P. Tagkalidis. "Oral Sodium Phosphate (Fleet) Is a
Superior Colonoscopy Preparation to Picopre (Sodium Picosulfate-Based
Preparation)." *Diseases of the Colon and Rectum* 49, no. 5 (2006): 616–20.

Hennessey, Rachel. "Living in Color: The Potential Dangers of Artificial Dyes."
Forbes, August 27, 2012. Accessed November 13, 2017. https://www.forbes.com
/sites/rachelhennessey/2012/08/27/living-in-color-the-potential-dangers-of
-artificial-dyes/#5574cd83107a.

The Smiling Man. "Artificial Colors in Food: Is FDA Certification Enough?" HubPages.

Last modified January 2, 2011. https://hubpages.com/food/GUIDE-TO-ARTIFICIAL
-FOOD-COLORINGS.

Adams, Mike. "Natural Consumer Products Found Contaminated with Cancer-
Causing 1,4-Dioxane in Groundbreaking Analysis Released by OCA." Organic
Consumers Association, March 15, 2008. Accessed November 13, 2017. https://
www.organicconsumers.org/news/natural-consumer-products-found
-contaminated-cancer-causing-14-dioxane-groundbreaking-analysis.

Environmental Working Group. "1,4-Dioxane." EWG's Skin Deep Cosmetics Database. Accessed November 13, 2017. https://www.ewg.org/skindeep/ingredient
/726331/1%2C4-DIOXANE/#.WgoivWiPKUl.

Environmental Working Group. "Fragrance." EWG's Skin Deep Cosmetics Database.
Accessed November 13, 2017. http://www.ewg.org/skindeep/ingredient/702512
/FRAGRANCE/#.Wgoi5miPKUl.

Environmental Working Group. "Polyethylene Glycol." EWG's Skin Deep Cosmetics
Database. Accessed November 13, 2017. http://www.ewg.org/skindeep
/ingredient/704983/POLYETHYLENE_GLYCOL/#.WgojCWiPKUl.

Pestano, Paul. "U.S. (Finally) Labels Formaldehyde 'Known Human Carcinogen.'"
EWG News and Analysis, June 13, 2011. Accessed November 20, 2017. https://
www.ewg.org/enviroblog/2011/06/us-finally-labels-formaldehyde-known
-human-carcinogen#.WgjAfxOPKu4.

Environmental Working Group. "Polyethelene Glycol." US Department of Health and
Human Services. "Chemical Information: Sodium Benzoate." Household Products Database. Accessed November 13, 2017. https://hpd.nlm.nih.gov/cgi-bin
/household/brands?tbl=chem&id=756&query=sodium+benzoate&searchas
=TblChemicals.

Mercola, Joseph. "Deadly and Dangerous Shampoos, Toothpastes, and Deter-
gents: Could 16,000 Studies Be Wrong About SLS?" Mercola.com, July 13, 2010.
Accessed November 13, 2017. https://articles.mercola.com/sites/articles
/archive/2010/07/13/sodium-lauryl-sulfate.aspx.

Congleton, Johanna. "Chemicals That Should Disappear from Cosmetics." EWG News
and Analysis, January 6, 2014. Accessed November 13, 2017. https://www.ewg.org
/enviroblog/2014/01/chemicals-should-disappear-cosmetics#.Wgoj_GiPKUm.

Artemis, Nadine. *Renegade Beauty*. Berkeley: North Atlantic Books, 2017.

Lee, Matilda, and Laura Sevier. "The A–Z of Eco Fashion." *Ecologist*, January 10, 2008. Accessed July 5, 2017. http://www.theecologist.org/green_green_living/clothing/269326/the_a_z_of_eco_fashion.html.

Greenpeace. *Toxic Threads: The Big Fashion Stitch-Up*. Amsterdam: Greenpeace International, 2012, pp. 13–14. http://www.greenpeace.org/international/Global/international/publications/toxics/Water%202012/ToxicThreads01.pdf.

Brown, H. S., D. R. Bishop, and C. A. Rowan. "The Role of Skin Absorption as a Route of Exposure for Volatile Organic Compounds (VOCs) in Drinking Water." *American Journal of Public Health* 74, no. 5 (1984): 479–84.

Centers for Disease Control and Prevention. "Skin Exposure and Effects." NIOSH, April 30, 2012. Accessed July 6, 2017. https://www.cdc.gov/niosh/topics/skin/default.html.

Luongo, Giovanna. "Chemicals in Textiles: A Potential Source for Human Exposure and Environmental Pollution." Doctoral thesis, Stockholm University, 2015. Accessed July 5, 2017. http://www.diva-portal.org/smash/get/diva2:850089/FULLTEXT02.pdf.

US Environmental Protection Agency. "Quinoline." September 2001. https://www.epa.gov/sites/production/files/2016–09/documents/quinoline.pdf.

Organic Trade Association. "Cotton and the Environment." April 2017. https://www.ota.com/advocacy/fiber-and-textiles/organic-cotton/cotton-and-environment.

Environmental Justice Foundation. *The Deadly Chemicals in Cotton*. Report written in collaboration with Pesticide Action Network UK. London: EJF, 2007. https://ejfoundation.org//resources/downloads/the_deadly_chemicals_in_cotton.pdf.

US Government Publishing Office. "Electronic Code of Federal Regulations: Part 205—National Organic Program, Subpart G." Accessed July 6, 2017. https://www.ecfr.gov/cgi-bin/text-idx?c=ecfr&SID=9874504b6f1025eb0e6b67cadf9d3b40&rgn=div6&view=text&node=7:3.1.1.9.32.7&idno=7#se7.3.205_1601.

Environmental Working Group. "Cheatsheet: Perfluorochemicals (PFCs)." EWG News and Analysis. April 29, 2008. http://www.ewg.org/enviroblog/2008/04/cheatsheet-perfluorochemicals-pfcs.

Greenpeace. *A Little Story About the Monsters in Your Closet*. Beijing: Greenpeace East Asia, January 2014. http://www.greenpeace.org/eastasia/Global/eastasia/publications/reports/toxics/2013/A%20Little%20Story%20About%20the%20Monsters%20In%20Your%20Closet%20-%20Report.pdf.

American Cancer Society. "What Causes Cancer?: Formaldehyde." Last modified May 23, 2014. https://www.cancer.org/cancer/cancer-causes/formaldehyde.html.

International Trade Administration. "Examples of Voluntary Formaldehyde Labeling Programs for Textile and Apparel Products." From US Government Accountability Office report *Formaldehyde in Textiles*, August 2010. http://web.ita.doc.gov/tacgi/eamain.nsf/ff5dd4f75c7795ea8525762500657ba8/cb13d7a21e9b08168525779800652683?OpenDocument.

Flynn, Valerie. "EU Countries Agree Textile Chemical Ban." *The Guardian*, July 21, 2015. https://www.theguardian.com/environment/2015/jul/21/eu-countries-agree-textile-chemical-ban.

Haydel, S. E., C. M. Remenih, and L. B. Williams. "Broad-Spectrum in Vitro Antibacterial Activities of Clay Minerals Against Antibiotic-Susceptible and Antibiotic-Resistant Bacterial Pathogens." *Journal of Antimicrobial Chemotherapy* 61, no. 2 (2008): 353–61.

St. George, Galina. *How Clays Work: Science and Applications of Clays and Clay-Like Minerals in Health and Beauty.* Self-pub., December 2016.

Carretero, M. I. "Clay Minerals and Their Beneficial Effects upon Human Health." *Applied Clay Science* 21, nos. 3–4 (2002): 155–63.

Price, Weston A. *Nutrition and Physical Degeneration: A Comparison of Primitive and Modern Diets and Their Effects.* Garsington, UK: Benediction Classics, 2010.

Bergaya, F., B. K. G. Theng, and G. Lagaly, eds. *Handbook of Clay Science.* 1st ed. Vol. 1 of *Developments in Clay Science.* Amsterdam: Elsevier, 2006.

Lapus, R. M. "Activated Charcoal for Pediatric Poisonings: The Universal Antidote?" *Current Opinion in Pediatrics* 19 (2007): 216–22. http://emergency.med.ufl.edu/files/2013/02/Activated-charcoal.pdf.

Holt Jr., L. E., and P. H. Holz. "The Black Bottle: A Consideration of the Role of Charcoal in the Treatment of Poisoning in Children." *Journal of Pediatrics* 63 (1963): 306–14.

Yatzidis, Hippocrates. "Activated Charcoal Rediscovered." Letter in *British Medical Journal* 4, no. 5831 (October 7, 1972): 51. http://www.bmj.com/content/4/5831/51.1.

University of Kentucky Center for Applied Energy Research. "History of Carbon." Accessed July 27, 2017. http://www.caer.uky.edu/carbon/history/carbonhistory.shtml.

Frolkis, V. V., V. G. Nikolaev, G. I. Paramonova, E. V. Shchorbitskaya, L. N. Bogats-kaya, A. S. Stupina, A. I. Kovtun, et al. "Effect of Enterosorption on Animal Lifespan." *Bimaterials, Artificial Cells, and Artificial Organs* 17, no. 3 (1989): 341–51.

Frolkis, V. V., V. G. Nikolaev, L. N. Bogatskaya, A. S. Stupina, E. V. Shchorbitskaya, A. I. Kovtun, G. I. Paramonova, et al. "Enterosorption in Prolonging Old Animal Lifespan." *Experimental Gerontology* 19, no. 4 (1984): 217–25.

Bird, James. *Vegetable Charcoal: Its Medicinal and Economic Properties, with Practical Remarks on Its Use in Chronic Affections of the Stomach and Bowels.* London: John Churchill, 1857.

Brightman, L., E. Weiss, A. M. Chapas, J. Karen, E. Hale, L. Bernstein, and R. G. Geronemus. "Improvement in Arm and Post-Partum Abdominal and Flank Sub-cutaneous Fat Deposits and Skin Laxity Using a Bipolar Radiofrequency, Infra-red, Vacuum, and Mechanical Massage Device." *Lasers in Surgery and Medicine* 41, no. 10 (2009): 791–98.

Liver Doctor. "Fat Cells and Toxins." August 29, 2016. Accessed August 9, 2017. https://www.liverdoctor.com/fat-cells-and-toxins/.

Chevrier, J., E. Dewailly, P. Ayotte, P. Mauriège, J. P. Després, and A. Tremblay. "Body Weight Loss Increases Plasma and Adipose Tissue Concentrations of Potentially Toxic Pollutants in Obese Individuals." *International Journal of Obesity and Related Disorders* 24, no. 10 (2000): 1272–78.

Beauty Factor 3: Nourish Cells

Thielitz, A., and H. Gollnick. "Topical Retinoids in Acne Vulgaris: Update on Efficacy and Safety." *American Journal of Clinical Dermatology* 9, no. 6 (2008): 369–81.

Darlenski, R., C. Surber, and J. W. Fluhr. "Topical Retinoids in the Management of Photodamaged Skin: From Theory to Evidence-Based Practical Approach." *British Journal of Dermatology* 163, no. 6 (2010): 1157–65.

Singh, M., and C. E. Griffiths. "The Use of Retinoids in the Treatment of Photoaging." *Dermatologic Therapy* 19, no. 5 (2006): 297–305.

Angelo, Giana. "Vitamin A and Skin Health." Linus Pauling Institute, Oregon State University, 2012. Accessed July 30, 2017. http://lpi.oregonstate.edu/mic/health -disease/skin-health/vitamin-A.

Pfahl, M. "Signal Transduction by Retinoid Receptors." *Skin Pharmacology: The Official Journal of the Skin Pharmacology Society* 6, suppl. 1 (1993): 8–16.

Wang, Z., M. Boudjelal, S. Kang, J. J. Voorhees, and G. J. Fisher. "Ultraviolet Irradiation of Human Skin Causes Functional Vitamin A Deficiency, Preventable by All-Trans Retinoic Acid Pre-Treatment." *Natural Medicine* 5, no. 4 (1999): 418–22.

Harnden, Thomas. "Fat-Soluble Vitamins." Lecture notes. Georgia Highlands College, February 22, 2013. Accessed August 6, 2017. http://www2.highlands.edu /academics/divisions/scipe/biology/faculty/harnden/2190/notes/9.htm.

Sharma, Ira. "19 Amazing Benefits of Cherries for Skin, Hair, and Health." StyleCraze. Last modified October 11, 2017. Accessed August 10, 2017. http://www .stylecraze.com/articles/top-10-health-benefits-of-cherries/#gref.

Duthie, S. J., and A. Hawdon. "DNA Instability (Strand Breakage, Uracil Misincorporation, and Defective Repair) Is Increased by Folic Acid Depletion in Human Lymphocytes in Vitro." *FASEB Journal* 12, no. 14 (1998): 1491–97.

Juhlin, L., and M. J. Olsson. "Improvement of Vitiligo After Oral Treatment with Vitamin B12 and Folic Acid and the Importance of Sun Exposure." *Acta Dermato-Venerologica* (Stockholm) 77, no. 6 (1997): 460–62.

Fischer, F., V. Achterberg, A. März, S. Puschmann, C. D. Rahn, V. Lutz, A. Krüger, et al. "Folic Acid and Creatinine Improve the Firmness of Human Skin in Vivo." *Journal of Cosmetic Dermatology* 10, no. 1 (2011): 15–23.

Singh, U., S. Devaraj, and I. Jialal. "Vitamin E, Oxidative Stress, and Inflammation." *Annual Review of Nutrition* 25 (2005): 151–74.

Nachbar, F., and H. C. Korting. "The Role of Vitamin E in Normal and Damaged Skin." *Journal of Molecular Medicine* (Berlin) 73, no. 1 (1995): 7–17.

Ehrlich, Melanie. "DNA Hypomethylation in Cancer Cells." *Epigenomics* 1, no. 2 (2009): 239–59.

Rhie, G., M. H. Shin, J. Y. Seo, W. W. Choi, K. H. Cho, K. H. Kim, K. C. Park, et al. "Aging- and Photoaging-Dependent Changes of Enzymic and Nonenzymic Antioxidants in the Epidermis and Dermis of Human Skin in Vivo." *Journal of Investigative Dermatology* 117, no. 5 (2001): 1212–17.

Ahmed, Arshi. "28 Amazing Benefits of Vitamin D for Skin, Hair, and Health." StyleCraze. Last modified September 19, 2017. Accessed August 10, 2017. http:// www.stylecraze.com/articles/vitamin-d-sources-deficiency-skin-hair-and -health-benefits/#gref.

Bowman, Joe, and Kristeen Cherney. "The 4 Best Vitamins for Your Skin." Health-line, August 1, 2016. Accessed August 10, 2017. https://www.healthline.com/health/4-best-vitamins-for-skin#vitamin-e4.

HomeRemediesforYou.com. "Vitamin K for Healthy and Beautiful Skin." Accessed August 10, 2017. http://www.home-remedies-for-you.com/vitamins/skin-vitamins/vitamin-k-for-skin.html.

Dillan, Jim. "Top 5 Vitamin K Benefits and the Best Sources." Health Ambition. Accessed August 10, 2017. https://www.healthambition.com/vitamin-k-benefits-best-sources/.

The Green Creator. "Why Is MSM My Beauty Mineral?" January 21, 2017. Accessed August 10, 2017. http://thegreencreator.com/why-is-msm-my-beauty-mineral/.

Goenka, Shruti. "16 Best Benefits of Magnesium for Skin, Hair, and Health." Style-Craze. Last modified September 19, 2017. Accessed August 10, 2017. http://www.stylecraze.com/articles/benefits-of-magnesium-for-skin-hair-and-health/#gref.

Home Remedy Hacks. "23 Proven Health and Beauty Benefits of Celery." June 26, 2015. Accessed August 10, 2017. https://www.homeremedyhacks.com/23-proven-health-and-beauty-benefits-of-celery/.

"The Skin Benefits of Selenium." *Canyon Ranch* (blog). Accessed August 10, 2017. https://www.canyonranch.com/blog/beauty/the-skin-benefits-of-selenium/.

Ashraf, R., R. A. Khan, and I. Ashraf. "Garlic (*Allium Sativum*) Supplementation with Standard Antidiabetic Agent Provides Better Diabetic Control in Type 2 Diabetes Patients." *Pakistan Journal of Pharmaceutical Sciences* 24, no. 4 (2011): 565–70.

Terry, Sarah. "The Use of Sulfur for Skin Care." Livestrong.com. Last modified July 18, 2017. Accessed August 10, 2017. http://www.livestrong.com/article/182861-the-use-of-sulfur-for-skin-care/.

Fernandez-Madrid, F., A. S. Prasad, and D. Oberleas. "Effect of Zinc Deficiency on Nucleic Acids, Collagen, and Noncollagenous Protein of the Connective Tissue." *Journal of Laboratory and Clinical Medicine* 82, no. 6 (1973): 951–61.

Gupta, M., V. Mahajan, K. S. Mehta, and P. S. Chauhan. "Zinc Therapy in Dermatology: A Review." *Dermatology Research and Practice* 2014 (2014): 709152.

Richie Jr., J. P., Y. Leutzinger, S. Parthasarathy, V. Malloy, N. Orentreich, and J. A. Zimmerman. "Methionine Restriction Increases Blood Glutathione and Longevity in F344 Rats." *FASEB Journal* 8, no. 15 (1994): 1302–7.

Swenson, Adam. "Glutathione: A Closer Look at the Master Antioxidant." *Natural Solutions Magazine,* June 30, 2013. Accessed August 5, 2017. http://d.natural solutionsmag.com/alternative-medicine/features/glutathione-closer-look -master-antioxidant.

Cascella, R., E. Evangelisti, M. Zampagni, M. Becatti, G. D'Adamio, A. Goti, G. Liguri, et al. "S-Linolenoyl Glutathione Intake Extends Life-Span and Stress Resistance via Sir-2.1 Upregulation in Caenorhabditis Elegans." *Free Radical Biology and Medicine* 73 (2014): 127–35.

Mercola, Joseph. "Your Practical Guide to Omega-3 Benefits and Supplementation." Mercola.com. Accessed August 10, 2017. https://articles.mercola.com/omega-3.aspx.

Graham, Blake. "Essential Fatty Acid Deficiency—Signs and Symptoms, Treating vs. Testing." ProHealth, July 7, 2009. Accessed August 10, 2017. http://www .prohealth.com/library/showarticle.cfm?libid=7564.

Better Health Thru Research. "316 Research Papers." Accessed August 10, 2017. http://www.betterhealththruresearch.com/340ResearchPapersChaga.htm.

Na, M., Y. H. Kim, B. S. Min, K. Bae, Y. Kamiryo, Y. Senoo, S. Yokoo, et al. "Cytoprotective Effect on Oxidative Stress and Inhibitory Effect on Cellular Aging of Uncaria Sinensis Havil." *Journal of Ethnopharmacology* 95, nos. 2–3 (2004): 127–32.

Howard, Diana. "Structural Changes Associated with Aging Skin." International Dermal Institute. Accessed November 20, 2017. http://www.dermalinstitute.com /us/library/11_article_Structural_Changes_AssociatAs_with_Aging_Skin.html.

Komaroff, Anthony. "What Happens to Our Skin as We Age?" Ask Doctor K., in association with Harvard Health Publications, July 22, 2014. Accessed November 20, 2017. https://www.askdoctork.com/happens-skin-age-201407226665.

US Geological Survey. "The Water in You." Water Science School. Accessed November 20, 2017. https://water.usgs.gov/edu/propertyyou.html.

Dermatology Review. "Dehydrated Skin." Accessed August 7, 2017. http://www .thedermreview.com/dehydrated-skin/.

Ousey, K., K. F. Cutting, A. A. Rogers, and M. G. Rippon. "The Importance of Hydration in Wound Healing: Reinvigorating the Clinical Perspective." *Journal of Wound Care* 25, no. 3 (2016): 122, 124–30.

Bella, J., B. Brodsky, and H. M. Berman. "Hydration Structure of a Collagen Peptide." *Structure* 3, no. 9 (1995): 893–906.

Wolfe, David. "Drink Water First Thing in the Morning for These 5 Reasons!" David Wolfe.com. Accessed August 15, 2017. https://www.davidwolfe.com/drink-water -first-morning-5-reasons/.

National Institute of Dental and Craniofacial Research. "The Story of Fluoridation." Last modified February 26, 2014. https://www.nidcr.nih.gov/OralHealth/Topics /Fluoride/TheStoryofFluoridation.htm.

Grandjean, P., and P. J. Landrigan. "Neurobehavioral Effects of Developmental Toxicity." *Lancet Neurology* 13, no. 3 (2014): 330–38.

National Research Council. "Fluoride in Drinking Water: A Scientific Review of EPA's Standards." Washington, DC: National Academies Press, 2006. https://www.nap .edu/catalog/11571/fluoride-in-drinking-water-a-scientific-review-of-epas -standards.

Centers for Disease Control and Prevention. "Lead." Last modified October 24, 2017. https://www.cdc.gov/nceh/lead/.

US Environmental Protection Agency. "Protect Your Family from Exposures to Lead." Last modified August 30, 2017. https://www.epa.gov/lead/protect-your -family-exposures-lead#water.

Curtis, Rick. "OA Guide to Water Purification." Princeton University, 1999. From *The Backpacker's Field Manual*. 1st ed. New York: Random House, 1998. http://www .princeton.edu/~oa/manual/water.shtml.

US Department of Health and Human Services. *Toxicology Profile for Polychlorinated Biphenyls (PCBs)*. November 2000. https://www.atsdr.cdc.gov/toxprofiles/tp17.pdf.

Oregon Health Authority Public Health Division. "Polychlorinated Biphenyls (PCBs) and Drinking Water." May 2015. http://www.oregon.gov/oha/ph/Healthy Environments/DrinkingWater/Monitoring/Documents/health/pcb.pdf.

World Health Organization. "Arsenic." Media Centre, June 2016. Last modified November 2017. http://www.who.int/mediacentre/factsheets/fs372/en/.

US Environmental Protection Agency. "Drinking Water Arsenic Rule History." Last modified November 2, 2016. https://www.epa.gov/dwreginfo/drinking-water -arsenic-rule-history.

Centers for Disease Control and Prevention. "Public Health Statement for Perchlorates." Agency for Toxic Substances and Disease Registry, September 2008. https://www.atsdr.cdc.gov/phs/phs.asp?id=892&tid=181.

US Environmental Protection Agency. "Technical Fact Sheet—Perchlorate." January 2014. https://www.epa.gov/sites/production/files/2014–03/documents/ffrro factsheet_contaminant_perchlorate_january2014_final.pdf.

Scheer, Roddy, and Doug Moss. "Perchlorate in Drinking Water Raises Health Concerns." EarthTalk. Reprinted in *Scientific American*, December 2012. Accessed July 9, 2017. https://www.scientificamerican.com/article/perchlorate-in-drinking -water/#.

Pesticide Action Network North America. "The DDT Story." Accessed July 9, 2017. http://www.panna.org/resources/ddt-story.

Geisz, H. N., R. M. Dickhut, M. A. Cochran, W. R. Fraser, and H. W. Ducklow. "Melting Glaciers: A Probable Source of DDT to the Antarctic Marine Ecosystem." *Environmental Science and Technology* 42, no. 11 (2008): 3958–62. http://pubs.acs .org/doi/pdf/10.1021/es702919n.

CalEPA Office of Environmental Health Hazard Assessment. "Glyphosate Listed Effective July 7, 2017, as Known to the State of California to Cause Cancer." Last modified June 26, 2017. Accessed July 10, 2017. https://oehha.ca.gov/proposition -65/crnr/glyphosate-listed-effective-july-7–2017-known-state-california-cause -cancer#_ftnref3.

US Geological Survey. "Glyphosate Herbicide Found in Many Midwestern Streams, Antibiotics Not Common." Last modified August 23, 2017. https://toxics.usgs .gov/highlights/glyphosate02.html.

The Detox Project. "Glyphosate in Food and Water." 2017. https://detoxproject.org /glyphosate-in-food-water/.

Fossel, Michael, Greta Blackburn, and Dave Woynarowski. *The Immortality Edge.* Hoboken, NJ: John Wiley, 2011, 140–46.

Blackburn, Elizabeth, and Elissa Epel. *The Telomere Effect: A Revolutionary Approach to Living Younger, Healthier, Longer.* New York: Grand Central, 2017.

Beauty Factor 4: Balance Hormones

Renew Health and Wellness. "Benefits of Testosterone for Women: The Case for Testosterone Replacement in Aging Women." Last modified January 23, 2017. Accessed August 19, 2017. https://www.renewmetoday.com/benefits-testosterone -women/.

American Thyroid Association. "General Information/Press Room." Accessed August 19, 2017. https://www.thyroid.org/media-main/about-hypo thyroidism/.

Kiersztan, A., N. Trojan, A. Tempes, P. Nalepa, J. Sitek, K. Winiarska, and M. Usarek. "DHEA Supplementation to Dexamethasone-Treated Rabbits Alleviates Oxidative Stress in Kidney-Cortex and Attenuates Albuminuria." *Journal of Steroid Biochemistry and Molecular Biology* 174 (2017): 17–26.

Daniell, H. W. "Potential Prevention by Oral DHEA of Superficial Tears in Elderly Atrophic Skin." *Journal of Steroid Biochemistry and Molecular Biology* 171 (2017): 155–56.

Ruan, Q., G. D'Onofrio, T. Wu, A. Greco, D. Sancarlo, and Z. Yu. "Sexual Dimorphism of Frailty and Cognitive Impairment: Potential Underlying Mechanisms (Review)." *Molecular Medicine Reports* 16, no. 3 (2017): 3023–33.

Kałużna-Czaplińska, J., P. Gątarek, S. Chirumbolo, M. S. Chartrand, and G. Bjørklund. "How Important Is Tryptophan in Human Health?" *Critical Reviews in Food Science and Nutrition* (August 11, 2017): 1–17 (online publ. before print).

Reich, A., and J. C. Szepietowski. "Mediators of Pruritus in Psoriasis." *Mediators of Inflammation* 2007 (2007): 64727.

Zero Breast Cancer. "Phthalates." Handout. Accessed July 7, 2017. https://www.niehs .nih.gov/research/supported/assets/docs/j_q/phthalates_the_everywhere _chemical_handout_508.pdf.

Johns, L. E., K. K. Ferguson, O. P. Soldin, D. E. Cantonwine, L. O. Rivera-González, L. V. Del Toro, A. M. Calafat, et al. "Urinary Phthalate Metabolites in Relation to Maternal Serum Thyroid and Sex Hormone Levels During Pregnancy: A Longitudinal Analysis." *Reproductive Biology and Endocrinology* 13, no. 4 (2015).

Centers for Disease Control and Prevention. "Phthalates." National Biomonitoring Program. Last modified December 23, 2016. Accessed November 20, 2017. https://www.cdc.gov/biomonitoring/phthalates_factsheet.html.

Environmental Working Group. "Analysis Finds Hormone Disruptor Used in Cosmetics in Nearly 50 Different Foods." News release. April 8, 2015. Accessed November 20, 2017. https://www.ewg.org/release/analysis-finds-hormone -disruptor-used-cosmetics-nearly-50-different-foods#.Wgn0oROPKu4.

Pestano, Paul. "Common Preservative in Personal Care Products Linked to Breast Cancer." EWG News and Analysis. November 24, 2015. Accessed November 20,

2017. https://www.ewg.org/enviroblog/2015/11/common-preservative-in -personal-care-products-linked-breast-cancer#.Wgn2HBOPKu4.

Sgobba, Christa. "Your Toothpaste Might Be Ruining Your Sperm." *Men's Health*, August 18, 2017. Accessed November 20, 2017. https://www.menshealth.com /health/parabens-and-sperm-quality.

US Food and Drug Administration. "Phthalates." Last modified December 5, 2013. Accessed July 7, 2017. https://www.fda.gov/Cosmetics/ProductsIngredients /Ingredients/ucm128250.htm.

Morgenstern, R., R. M. Whyatt, B. J. Insel, A. M. Calafat, X. Liu, V. A. Rauh, J. Herbstman, et al. "Phthalates and Thyroid Function in Preschool Age Children: Sex Specific Associations." *Environment International* 106 (2017): 11–18.

Environmental Working Group. "Teen Girls' Body Burden of Hormone-Altering Cosmetics Chemicals: Cosmetics Chemicals of Concern." September 24, 2008. Accessed November 20, 2017. https://www.ewg.org/research/teen-girls-body -burden-hormone-altering-cosmetics-chemicals/cosmetics-chemicals-concern #.WgnuaxOPKu5.

Mercola, Joseph. "Women Beware: Most Feminine Hygiene Products Contain Toxic Ingredients." Mercola.com, May 22, 2013. Accessed November 20, 2017. https:// articles.mercola.com/sites/articles/archive/2013/05/22/feminine-hygiene -products.aspx.

Zerbe, Leah. "BPA and Skin Exposure: Chemical Easily Moves from Receipts into Your Body." Rodale Wellness, February 27, 2014. Accessed July August 19, 2017. https://www.rodalewellness.com/health/bpa-and-skin-exposure.

Liu, J., J. Li, Y. Wu, Y. Zhao, F. Luo, S. Li, L. Yang, et al. "Bisphenol A Metabolites and Bisphenol S in Paired Maternal and Cord Serum." *Environmental Science and Technology* 51, no. 4 (2017): 2456–63.

Mercola, Joseph. "How BPA and BPS Are Making People Sick." Mercola.com, February 22, 2017. Accessed November 20, 2017. https://articles.mercola.com/sites/articles /archive/2017/02/22/bpa-bps-making-people-sick.aspx.

Leonard, Jayne. "10 Hidden Sources of Toxins Lurking in Your Kitchen and Pantry." Natural Living Ideas, September 8, 2015. Accessed July 30, 2017. http://www .naturallivingideas.com/hidden-sources-of-toxins-in-your-kitchen/.

Main, Emily. "The Top 12 Worst Chemicals in Your Home." Rodale Wellness.

Accessed July 30, 2017. https://www.rodalewellness.com/health/endocrine-disruptors-list/learn-more/slide/1.

Kristoffer, Heidi. "7 Common Hidden Toxins Hanging Out in Your Kitchen That You Should Know." Natural News Blogs, October 3, 2014. Accessed July 30, 2017. https://www.naturalnewsblogs.com/7-common-hidden-toxins-hanging-kitchen-know/.

Dodson, R. E., M. Nishioka, L. J. Standley, L. J. Perovich, J. G. Brody, and R. A. Rude. "Endocrine Disruptors and Asthma-Associated Chemicals in Consumer Products." *Environmental Health Perspectives* 120, no. 7 (2012): 935–43.

Patisaul, H. B., and W. Jefferson. "The Pros and Cons of Phytoestrogens." *Frontiers in Neuroendocrinology* 31, no. 4 (2010): 400–19.

Hsiao, Y. H., S. Y. Hsia, Y. C. Chan, and J. F. Hsieh. "Complex Coacervation of Soy Proteins, Isoflavones, and Chitosan." *Molecules* 22, no. 6 (2017).

Silva, L. A., A. A. Ferraz Carbonel, A. R. B. De Moraes, R. S. Simões, G. R. D. S. Sasso, L. Goes, W. Nunes, et al. "Collagen Concentration on the Facial Skin of Postmenopausal Women After Topical Treatment with Estradiol and Genistein: A Randomized Double-Blind Controlled Trial." *Gynecological Endocrinology* 33, no. 11 (2017): 845–48.

Patisaul, H. B. "Endocrine Disruption of Vasopressin Systems and Related Behaviors." *Frontiers in Endocrinology* (Lausanne) 8 (2017): 134.

European Commission Health and Consumer Protection Directorate-General. *Opinion of the Scientific Committee on Veterinary Measures Relating to Public Health on Review of Previous SCVPH Opinions of 30 April 1999 and 3 May 2000 on the Potential Risks to Human Health from Hormone Residues in Bovine Meat and Meat Products.* Retrieved November 21, 2012. https://ec.europa.eu/food/sites/food/files/safety/docs/cs_meat_hormone-out50_en.pdf.

Biro, F. M., M. P. Galvez, L. C. Greenspan, P. A. Succop, N. Vangeepuram, S. M. Pinney, S. Teitelbaum, et al. "Pubertal Assessment Method and Baseline Characteristics in a Mixed Longitudinal Study of Girls." *Pediatrics* (August 2010).

Daubenmier, J., D. Hayden, V. Chang, and E. Epel. "It's Not What You Think, It's How You Relate to It: Dispositional Mindfulness Moderates the Relationship Between Psychological Distress and the Cortisol Awakening Response." *Psychoneuroendocrinology* 48 (2014): 11–18.

Phillips, K. M., M. H. Antoni, S. C. Lechner, B. B. Blomberg, M. M. Llabre, E. Avisar, S. Glück, et al. "Stress Management Intervention Reduces Serum Cortisol and Increases Relaxation During Treatment for Nonmetastatic Breast Cancer." *Psychosomatic Medicine* 70, no. 9 (2008): 1044–49.

Tait, Janine. "Hormones and the Skin." Beautymagonline.com. Accessed August 26, 2017. http://www.beautymagonline.com/sample-pages/1193-hormones-and-their-effect-onthe-skin-2.

Goenka, Shruti. "Estrogen Benefits for Skin, Hair, and Health." StyleCraze. Last modified November 2, 2017. Accessed August 26, 2017. http://www.stylecraze.com/articles/estrogen-benefits-for-skin-hair-and-health/#gref.

Centers for Disease Control and Prevention. "1 in 3 Adults Don't Get Enough Sleep." News release. February 18, 2016. Accessed August 10, 2017. https://www.cdc.gov/media/releases/2016/p0215-enough-sleep.html.

Berger, Jody. "Ayurvedic Time and Balanced Sleep." *VPK by Maharishi Ayurveda* (blog), November 24, 2015. Accessed August 10, 2017. http://www.mapi.com/blog/ayurvedic-time-and-balanced-sleep.html.

Harding, Mary. "Pituitary Function Tests." Patient, August 3, 2015. Accessed August 20, 2017. https://patient.info/doctor/pituitary-function-tests#.

National Sleep Foundation. "Normal Sleep." In *The Sleep Disorders*, 2017. http://sleepdisorders.sleepfoundation.org/chapter-1-normal-sleep/the-physiology-of-sleep-the-endocrine-system-sleep/.

Spiegel, K., E. Tasali, P. Penev, and E. Van Cauter. "Brief Communication: Sleep Curtailment in Healthy Young Men Is Associated with Decreased Leptin Levels, Elevated Ghrelin Levels, and Increased Hunger and Appetite." *Annals of Internal Medicine* 141, no. 11 (2004): 846–50.

Kloss, J. D., M. L. Perlis, J. A. Zamzow, E. J. Culnan, and C. R. Garcia. "Sleep, Sleep Disturbance, and Fertility in Women." *Sleep Medicine Reviews* 22 (2015): 78–87.

Vermeulen, A., J. M. Kaufman, J. P. Deslypere, and G. Thomas. "Attenuated Luteinizing Hormone (LH) Pulse Amplitude but Normal LH Pulse Frequency, and Its Relation to Plasma Androgens in Hypogonadism of Obese Men." *Journal of Clinical Endocrinology and Metabolism* 76, no. 5 (1993): 1140–46.

Osansky, Eric. "This Is How Sleep Deprivation Can Lead to a Thyroid Condition." Natural Endocrine Solutions, May 19, 2011. Accessed August 20, 2017. http://www.naturalendocrinesolutions.com/archives/this-is-how-sleep-deprivation-can-lead-to-a-thyroid-condition/.

Pereira Jr., J. C., and M. L. Andersen. "The Role of Thyroid Hormone in Sleep Deprivation." *Medical Hypotheses* 82, no. 3 (2014): 350–55.

Beauty Factor 5: Overcome Stress

Statista. "Size of the Global Hair Care Market from 2012 to 2024 (in Billion US Dollars)." August 2017. Accessed November 20, 2017. https://www.statista.com/statistics/254608/global-hair-care-market-size/.

Epel, E. S., E. H. Blackburn, J. Lin, F. S. Dhabhar, N. E. Adler, J. D. Morrow, and R. M. Cawthon. "Accelerated Telomere Shortening in Response to Life Stress." *Proceedings of the National Academy of Sciences of the United States of America* 101, no. 49 (2004): 17312–15.

Slezak, Michael. "Stress May Cause Women's Brains to Age Prematurely." *New Scientist*, July 26, 2012. Accessed August 7, 2017. https://www.newscientist.com/article/dn22107-stress-may-cause-womens-brains-to-age-prematurely/.

Segerstrom, S. C., and G. E. Miller. "Psychological Stress and the Human Immune System: A Meta-Analytic Study of 30 Years of Inquiry." *Psychological Bulletin* 130, no. 4 (2004): 601–30.

Kiecolt-Glaser, J. K., D. L. Habash, C. P. Fagundes, R. Andridge, J. Peng, W. B. Malarkey, and M. A. Belury. "Daily Stressors, Past Depression, and Metabolic Responses to High-Fat Meals: A Novel Path to Obesity." *Biological Psychiatry* 77, no. 7 (2015): 653–60.

Calabrese, F., R. Molteni, G. Racagni, and M. A. Riva. "Neuronal Plasticity: A Link Between Stress and Mood Disorders." *Psychoneuroendocrinology* 34, suppl. 1 (2009): S208–16.

Son, H., M. Banasr, M. Choi, S. Y. Chae, P. Licznerski, B. Lee, B. Voleti, et al. "Neuritin Produces Antidepressant Actions and Blocks the Neuronal and Behavioral Deficits Caused by Chronic Stress." *Proceedings of the National Academy of Sciences of the United States of America* 109, no. 28 (2012): 11378–83. http://www.pnas.org/content/109/28/11378.abstract.

Bodenmann, G., T. Ledermann, D. Blattner, and C. Galluzzo. "Associations Among Everyday Stress, Critical Life Events, and Sexual Problems." *Journal of Nervous and Mental Disease* 194, no. 7 (2006): 494–501.

Saitta, P., C. E. Cook, J. L. Messina, R. Brancaccio, B. C. Wu, S. K. Grekin, and J. Holland. "Is There a True Concern Regarding the Use of Hair Dye and Malignancy

Development? A Review of the Epidemiological Evidence Relating Personal Hair Dye Use to the Risk of Malignancy." *Journal of Clinical and Aesthetic Dermatology* 6, no. 1 (2013): 39–46.

Vazirian, M., M. A. Faramarzi, S. E. Ebrahimi, H. R. Esfahani, N. Samadi, S. A. Hosseini, A. Asghari, et al. "Antimicrobial Effect of the Lingzhi or Reishi Medicinal Mushroom, *Ganoderma Lucidum* (Higher Basidiomycetes) and Its Main Compounds." *International Journal of Medicinal Mushrooms* 16, no. 1 (2014): 77–84.

Zhang, W., J. Tao, X. Yang, Z. Yang, L. Zhang, H. Liu, K. Wu, et al. "Antiviral Effects of Two *Ganoderma Lucidum* Triterpenoids Against Enterovirus 71 Infection." *Biochemical and Biophysical Research Communications* 449, no. 3 (2014): 307–12.

Chiu, H. F., H. Y. Fu, Y. Y. Lu, Y. C. Han, Y. C. Shen, K. Venkatakrishnan, O. Golovinskaia, et al. "Triterpenoids and Polysaccharide Peptides-Enriched *Ganoderma Lucidum*: A Randomized, Double-Blind Placebo-Controlled Crossover Study of Its Antioxidation and Hepatoprotective Efficacy in Healthy Volunteers." *Pharmaceutical Biology* 55, no. 1 (2017): 1041–46.

Akihisa, T., Y. Nakamua, M. Tagata, H. Tokuda, K. Yasukawa, E. Uchiyama, T. Suzuki, et al. "Anti-Inflammatory and Anti-Tumor-Promoting Effects of Triterpine Acids and Sterols from the Fungus *Ganoderma Lucidum*." *Chemistry and Biodiversity* 4, no. 2 (2007): 224–31.

Wu, H., S. Tang, Z. Huang, Q. Zhou, P. Zhang, and Z. Chen. "Hepatoprotective Effects and Mechanisms of Action of Triterpenoids from Lingzhi or Reishi Medicinal Mushroom *Ganoderma Lucidum* (Agaricomycetes) on α-Amanitin-Induced Liver Injury in Mice." *International Journal of Medicinal Mushrooms* 18, no. 9 (2016): 841–50.

Chen, L. W., L. Y. Horng, C. L. Wu, H. C. Sung, and R. T. Wu. "Activating Mitochondrial Regulator PGC-1α Expression by Astrocytic NGF Is a Therapeutic Strategy for Huntington's Disease." *Neuropharmacology* 63, no. 4 (2012): 719–32.

Kim, J. W., H. I. Kim, J. H. Kim, O. C. Kwon, E. S. Son, C. S. Lee, and Y. J. Park. "Effects of Ganodermanondiol, a New Melanogenesis Inhibitor from the Medicinal Mushroom *Ganoderma Lucidum*." *International Journal of Molecular Science* 17, no. 11 (2016).

Jin, M., Y. Zhu, D. Shao, K. Zhao, C. Xu, Q. Li, H. Yang, et al. "Effects of Polysaccharide from Mycelia of *Ganoderma Lucidum* on Intestinal Barrier Functions of Rats." *International Journal of Biological Macromolecules* 94, pt. A (2017): 1–9.

INDEX

ABOUT THE AUTHORS

David "Avocado" Wolfe is a highly sought after health and longevity speaker with a passion for integrating superfoods and superherbs into everyday living, fueling his dynamic desire to create "the best day ever."

Leading the charge for radiant health and natural living by sparking a worldwide lifestyle movement into superfoods, superherbs, living spring water, and raw chocolate, he shares information gleaned from years of collegiate study, as well as hands-on experience as an organic farmer and beekeeper.

David has traveled around the world to twenty-nine countries, hosting over three thousand live events and retreats, where he champions the ideals of spending time in nature, living sustainably, maintaining a positive mental attitude, and eating the best food ever. A nutritional consultant to celebrities, elite athletes, and parents and children alike, he empowers everyone to take the responsibility for healthy living into their own hands.

David is the celebrity spokesperson for one of America's leading kitchen appliances: the NUTRiBULLET™. His Facebook page (www .facebook.com/DavidAvocadoWolfe) and Facebook videos and posts reach millions of people each week around the world with succinct, powerful inspirational quotes, news, health information, and education. David's Facebook fan base is over 12 million strong, making his influence one of the most widely commented on, clicked on, and shared in the world.

David is the visionary founder and president of the award-winning nonprofit charity the Fruit Tree Planting Foundation (www.ftpf.org). FTPF has a mission to alleviate world hunger by planting 18 million food-bearing trees on earth.

Author of the bestselling books *Eating for Beauty*, *The Sunfood Diet Success System*, *Naked Chocolate*, *Superfoods: The Food and Medicine of the Future*, *Chaga: King of the Medicinal Mushrooms*, *Longevity Now*, *The Longevity Now Program*, *The Adrenal Health Program*, and *The Mega Immunity Program*, he has also appeared in numerous breakthrough documentaries and films including *Food Matters*, *Hungry for Change*, and *Raw for Life*. David has appeared on hundreds of broadcast programs and in print media around the world including CNN's *Anderson Cooper 360°*, *Men's Health*, *Woman's Day*, and *Vegetarian Times*. David is one of the lead educators at the Longevity Now® Conference, the Women's Wellness Conference™, the Institute of Integrative Nutrition, and the Body-Mind Institute.

R. A. Gauthier is the creator, director, emcee, and speaker at both the Longevity Now® Conference and the Women's Wellness Conference® events held in Southern California, where for over a decade millions of people have learned the latest in cutting-edge alternative health information.

She has shared the stage with top health visionaries including Dr. Daniel Amen, John Robbins, Dr. Sara Gottfried, Dr. Joel Fuhrman, Dr. Joseph Mercola, Caroline Myss, and Marianne Williamson, as well as being a featured host on the *David Wolfe Podcast*™ with more than six million listeners.

R. A. Gauthier is also the cocreator and writer of the bestselling Longevity Now Program, as well as the creator and producer of several other successful DVD health programs with David Wolfe. She is the cofounder of Longevity Warehouse, an online wellness specialty site offering the highest-integrity organic and wild-crafted foods from the cleanest sources available on earth.

She currently lives in Southern California with her husband and feisty five-year-old daughter.